SO-EIU-477

A
MANUAL
OF
NEWBORN
MEDICINE

Edited by: GERARD VAN LEEUWEN, M. D.

Professor and Chairman,
Department of Pediatrics,
University of Nebraska
College of Medicine,
Omaha, Nebraska

NO LONGER THE PROPERTY
OF THE
UNIVERSITY OF R. I. LIBRARY

YEAR BOOK MEDICAL PUBLISHERS, INC.
35 East Wacker Drive · Chicago

Copyright © 1973 by Year Book Medical Publishers, Inc.
All rights reserved. No part of this publication may be reproduced, stored in a retrieval system, or transmitted, in any form or by any means, electronic, mechanical, photocopying, recording, or otherwise, without prior written permission from the publisher. Printed in the United States of America.

Library of Congress Catalog Card Number: 72-88827
International Standard Book Number: 0-8151-8968-0

18857

Dedicated To

DR. BOB JACKSON

Chairman of Pediatrics at the University of Missouri, who was always able to overlook my shortcomings and point out my strengths. Six of the authors of this book were his residents, fellows or colleagues.

Preface

This book is designed for the practitioner and the student of general pediatrics.

This is a "think and do" book, emphasizing the "do." It grew from a handout for pediatric house officers and students, who, although they were good thinkers, found themselves frequently unprepared to do something about the emergency of the neonate.

We hope that some of our little patients' lives (and brains) will be preserved as a result of the contents of this book. We also hope good practitioners and students will explore the subjects in greater depth than is possible here.

CONTRIBUTING AUTHORS

GEORGE BAKER, M.D.

Associate Professor, Department of Pediatrics, and Director of Newborn Services, University Hospitals, Iowa City, Iowa

RICHARD GUTHRIE, M.D.

Associate Professor of Pediatrics, University of Missouri School of Medicine, Columbia, Missouri

ELIZABETH JAMES, M.D.

Assistant Professor of Pediatrics and of Obstetrics and Gynecology; Director of Newborn Services, University of Missouri School of Medicine, Columbia, Missouri

JOHN JONES, M.D.

Professor of Anesthesia and Executive Associate Dean, Medical College of Virginia, Richmond, Virginia

JOHN LUKENS, M.D.

Associate Professor of Pediatrics, Drew Institute Medical College, Los Angeles, California

ROBERT MESSER, M.D.

Professor and Chairman, Department of Obstetrics and Gynecology, University of Nebraska College of Medicine, Omaha, Nebraska

PAUL MOORING, M.D.

Professor, Department of Pediatrics, University of Nebraska College of Medicine, Omaha, Nebraska

GERARD VAN LEEUWEN, M.D.

Professor and Chairman, Department of Pediatrics University of Nebraska College of Medicine, Omaha, Nebraska

HOBART WILTSE, M.D.

Associate Professor, Department of Pediatrics, University of Nebraska College of Medicine, Omaha, Nebraska

YOSHIO (GEORGE) MIYAZAKI, M.D.

Assistant Professor and Director of Newborn Services, University of Nebraska College of Medicine, Omaha, Nebraska

Contents

Contents

A MANUAL OF
NEWBORN MEDICINE

CHAPTER 1

Maternal Factors in Newborn Medicine

ROBERT MESSER, M.D.

It is obvious that newborn care will be facilitated if, at the earliest possible time, risk factors can be identified and, ideally, overcome. Therefore, one should embrace the concept that newborn care begins before birth. This means that there should be a team approach to newborn care between obstetrician and pediatrician. But in the case of a primary physician who assumes responsibility for both mother and child, maternal factors which influence newborn medicine should be known and understood as thoroughly as possible. For example, he should know that in most cases, if a newborn is going to require intensive care in a newborn intensive-care center, the best incubator for his transportation is the mother.

In a text of limited scope, is impossible to detail all of these maternal factors. Furthermore, the medical literature is replete with conflicting viewpoints on the management of maternal complications. Therefore, in an effort to be concise, a series of didactic protocols will be outlined. These represent guidelines of a particular obstetric department for the management of certain obstetric problems. It is undeniable that deviations from these protocols may represent good medical care in individual cases. It is also undeniable that contrary viewpoints may be legitimate, and it is probable that future modification will be necessary.

GENERAL GUIDELINES

Routine Care

Ideally, pregnancy should occur when medical conditions are most favorable. This means that family planning for ideal pregnancy timing is important, as are preconceptional and interconceptional care. When pregnancy occurs, early and adequate prenatal care are important. Standard laboratory tests are, initially, hemoglobin (hematocrit), serology, blood type and Rh, and irregular antibody screening. Urine is checked for sugar and protein at each visit. (Individualized laboratory tests will be described later.) Weight, blood pressure and fundal growth are assessed at each visit. Visits are monthly until 28 weeks' gestation, biweekly until 36 and weekly thereafter. The hemoglobin test is repeated at 36 weeks.

Nutrition

About 24 pounds is suggested as the allowable weight gain in pregnancy. Underweight gravidas should not be too restricted in caloric intake. The most important component of the diet probably is protein. The minimum daily requirement of protein during pregnancy, according to the Committee on Maternal Nutrition of the National Research Council, is 65 Gm./day; during lactation, 75 Gm./day is recommended. The most important mineral supplement is iron, and the most important vitamin supplement probably is folic acid. Most U.S. prenatal vitamin supplements seem adequate to prevent iron and folic acid deficiency if these conditions do not pre-exist. For further nutritional details, the cited publication of the council (see Suggested Readings) is an excellent source.

Activity

Usual activity is not contraindicated in normal pregnancy, nor is swimming, tub baths and the like. Sexual intercourse at any stage of pregnancy is interdicted only in the presence of ruptured membranes, vaginal bleeding or excessive discomfort. The unusual sexual practice of blowing air into the vagina with some pressure is contraindicated during pregnancy: it may be fatal. Travel should be undertaken with caution during the first 8 weeks and the last 8 weeks—not because travel per se may be harmful, but because medical care may be unavailable when needed.

PREMATURITY

Unfortunately, at this time most instances of prematurity are unpredictable and unpreventable. However, certain guidelines may be helpful.

Known Prematurity

If a history of premature spontaneous termination of pregnancy (repeated episodes, particularly) is elicited, efforts should be made to find a treatable cause. Careful over-all medical evaluation is indicated. Hysterosalpingography as part of interconceptional care may identify uterine anomalies, submucous myomas or endometrial polyps. To detect these same conditions the uterus should be explored manually after a premature delivery. If an incompetent cervix is suspected from the history, the cervix should be examined weekly or every other week during the middle trimester. In a typical history of incompetent cervix there are repeated second-trimester pregnancy losses with very short labors and the absence of pre- or intrapartum bleeding.

Medical Control of Premature Labor

Unfortunately, at the present time we lack an agent which will consistently arrest established premature labor. The best results have been obtained with the use of isoxsuprine hydrochloride (Vasodilan). It is initially administered by dilute intravenous infusion, then orally if contractions cease. We do not have a standard dose, because each patient differs in her response to this drug, which must be used with great caution. The dose is titrated against uterine irritability and against blood pressure and pulse. The principal side effects are hypotension and tachycardia. Contraindications are vaginal bleeding, ruptured membranes, cervical dilatation greater than 3 cm., hypotension or tachycardia.

Surgical Prevention of Prematurity

Many surgical procedures have been devised to correct incompetency of the cervical os. Our guidelines are as follows:

1. The procedure is done between weeks 12 and 29 of gestation.

2. The least traumatic procedure is usually used, such as a purse-string, nonabsorbable suture, with minimal dissection—a procedure similar to the one described by McDonald.

3. At the onset of labor or at fetal maturity, the suture is removed and vaginal delivery is anticipated.

4. Rupture of membranes in the presence of a cervical suture is regarded as a dangerous situation from the standpoint of infection. Measures should be taken to effect delivery. (See section on premature rupture of the membranes.)

5. After 28 weeks the procedure itself may initiate premature labor, and bed rest is felt to be preferable to surgery.

Avoidance of "Elective Prematurity"

Pregnancy is often terminated before term for medical reasons, such as maternal diabetes, or for elective repeat cesarean section. It is extremely important to deliver a mature baby, if possible, when preterm delivery is elected. The following are our current methods of determining fetal maturity:

1. Early detection of pregnancy, preferably by the time of the second missed menstrual period.

2. Careful recording of the date of quickening. This is a rough guide, but generally if one adds 22 weeks to the quickening date of a multiparous patient and 20 weeks to that of a primigravida, the due date is approximated.

3. Careful note of the first audibility of fetal heart tones. These are generally heard at about 20 weeks with a standard head-type fetuscope.

4. A fundal height exceeding 28 cm. by calipers usually indicates size compatible with fetal maturity.

5. Careful clinical estimation of fetal size by more than one examiner. Success by this method will be directly proportional to the number and the experience of the examiners, but the method remains fallible.

6. X-ray. The clearly visible appearance of distal femoral epiphyses on a lateral film of the abdomen practically assures fetal development compatible with fetal maturity. A heavily calcified skull is a helpful sign. So is a well-developed fetal fat line; but it should be remembered that if the mother is diabetic, a well-developed fetal fat line may not indicate maturity: babies of diabetic mothers have excessive fat.

7. Amniocentesis. Increasing emphasis has been placed in recent years on the analysis of amniotic fluid with respect to determination of fetal maturity. Such parameters as total bilirubin, Nile blue sulfate staining and osmolality have been described as being helpful. In our experience the level of creatinine in amniotic fluid has been the most consistent indicator of fetal maturity. If the level exceeds 2 mg./100 ml., the baby is probably mature; if the level is less than 1.5 mg./100 ml., the baby is probably immature. At the present time the measurement of phospholipids in amniotic fluid as an indicator of fetal lung maturity is of interest. Our experience is limited, but it appears from preliminary results that the work of Gluck et al. can be reproduced. If the amount of lecithin in amniotic fluid significantly exceeds the amount of sphingomyelin, hyaline membrane disease appears unlikely. The true value of this test needs further explication.

Over-all, the fewest errors will be made if all of these methods are used in a co-ordinated way. In other words, one should not rely on a single determinant.

Multiple Gestation

Prematurity represents the greatest threat to the products of multiple gestation. Labor complications may also be significant. This has led to the following guidelines for the management of multiple gestation:

1. Suspected multiple gestation is confirmed by x-ray.

2. Bed rest after 30 weeks' gestation is encouraged, in an attempt to decrease the incidence of prematurity. This can be done at home, if the patient is co-operative.

3. At the onset of labor an intravenous infusion is started in anticipation of complications, such as postpartum hemorrhage.

4. The first baby is delivered with regional anesthesia, preferably. General anesthesia should be available in case intrauterine manipulation is required.

5. Adequate care for the newborn is scheduled in advance. This includes preparedness for prematurity and for the intertwin transfusion syndrome, in which one newborn is anemic and the other is plethoric—either condition being dangerous. Also, the malnourished twin is subject to hypoglycemia.

PREMATURE RUPTURE OF THE MEMBRANES

The management of the patient with rupture of the membranes prior to onset of labor is controversial. Our guidelines are as follows:

1. Confirm rupture of the membranes. Usually this is easy: there is a characteristic history of a gush of fluid, continued leaking and a positive nitrazine test. In doubtful cases, ambulation with collection of fluid on a perineal pad may be helpful. At present there is no consistent enthusiasm for other methods, because of ambiguous results in the most difficult cases. When the physician is in doubt, the patient must have individual management which considers her reliability, multiple risk factors, and the like.

2. If the baby is estimated to weigh less than 2,000 Gm., the patient is dismissed from the hospital, instructed to take her temperature twice a day, abstain from intercourse and douching, and continue outpatient visits. She is instructed to report any fever immediately. One hopes that infection, if it does occur, will be caused by a nonresistant, nonhospital organism.

3. If the patient is unreliable or is unable to adequately follow directions, she is hospitalized.

4. If the baby is estimated to weigh more than 2,000 Gm. and if labor does not ensue within 24 hours, labor is induced with dilute intravenous oxytocin. The temperature should be recorded every 2 hours.

5. The use of cesarean section for this condition is justified in some circumstances—particularly if infection supervenes, for then it is felt that prompt delivery is imperative. This is highly individualized, as is the management of abnormal presentations and multiple pregnancies complicated by premature rupture of the membranes.

6. Once the patient's status with regard to position, station and cervical dilatation is clarified, no further vaginal examinations are done in the absence of labor. Even when labor ensues, these examinations should be limited.

7. Prophylactic antibiotics are not used, unless prolonged labor and rupture of the membranes coexist.

PLACENTAL INSUFFICIENCY
(Intrauterine Growth Retardation)

It is difficult to arrive at a uniform plan of management for this complex problem, but a reasonable set of guidelines can be offered:

1. Placental insufficiency sometimes occurs in pregnancies that continue beyond the expected date of confinement; but it is important to recognize that postdatism is not synonymous with placental insufficiency. We believe, therefore, that when spontaneous labor does not occur after an expected date, this in itself does not constitute a medical indication for the induction of labor.

2. Clinical signs of placental insufficiency are several. Failure to gain weight near the end of pregnancy or actual loss of weight at that time is characteristic. The use of diuretics or the presence of edema may confuse this sign. Failure of fetal growth may be reflected by decreasing size of the uterus or decreasing abdominal girth. Whether this reflects lack of fetal growth alone or a decrease in the volume of amniotic fluid may be immaterial, because in severe cases the two often seem to coincide. In many cases clinical situations which may be associated with increased risk of growth retardation are recognizable; these include the hypertensive disorders, diabetes and maternal renal disease.

3. If placental insufficiency is suspected, an assessment of the feto-placental unit should be carried out. In our hands the most reliable laboratory index has been measurement of maternal urinary excretion of estriol. The amount found in the maternal urine is dependent primarily upon the function of the placenta and an intact fetal adrenal-pituitary axis. Obstetric literature abounds with testimony to the fact that this test is usually a reliable indicator of fetal welfare; however, the value of the test in actually improving perinatal survival has not been proved beyond a doubt. With the method of extraction used in our laboratories, values of less than 20 mg./24 hours are likely to indicate fetal distress. Serial values, obtained at intervals of 3 to 5 days, are more useful than single determinations. One must know the normal values and limitations of the test for each laboratory.

Another worthwhile test is the determination of serum heat-stable alkaline phosphatase, an enzyme primarily of the placenta. The determination is simple and relatively inexpensive; for details see the Suggested Readings. In our experience this test correlates with estriol determinations in about 66% of cases. Because this is a measurement of an unknown placental function, it is not surprising that it does not always correlate with estriol excretion. For example, a condition such as maternal hypoglycemia might threaten the fetus yet not affect placental function. Conversely, placental damage may occur, as in an infarct, but the fetus may not be threatened, if adequate placental reserve exists.

The work of Hon and others had delineated the response of the fetal heart to distress. Thus it is possible to "test" fetal well-being by subjecting the fetus to the stress of artificially induced uterine contractions and monitoring the fetal heart beat. If the rate slows in synchrony with the uterine contraction, this is interpreted as physiologic. However, if fetal bradycardia persists after the contraction and there is a delay in return to the precontraction rate, uteroplacental insufficiency should be suspected. This "late deceleration" pattern or a sustained bradycardia may signify fetal jeopardy: placental function may not be adequate for the fetus to survive normal labor.

4. At whatever point the evaluation of the fetus indicates that its survival chances would be greater outside the uterus, intervention is indicated. At this stage of medical knowledge, such an end point cannot be established from a set of rules. The matter requires the finest judgment, the weighing of clinical and laboratory parameters in each case, and the intellectual honesty to admit the great ignorance of medical science in the field of intrauterine diagnosis.

INFECTIONS

Only the most important maternal infections involving fetal welfare can be considered here. Again, certain arbitrary guidelines have been established.

Rubella

Maternal rubella infection can be accurately identified in the laboratory. Two questions usually need to be answered: Is the patient immune? Has the patient had rubella at a recent point in time (usually following exposure)? A hemagglutination-inhibition (HI) titer of less than 1:10 is interpreted as meaning that little immunity exists—that most probably there has not been a prior infection. Tissue immunity (as opposed to circulating immunity) cannot be accurately measured. For the question of recent infection, two blood samples are drawn, 2 weeks apart. The sera are frozen and are run at the same time; thus they serve to control each other. A two-tube rise (four dilution) is taken to imply recent infection. Complement-fixation tests are likely to be positive with recent infection, negative with old infections.

The following are suggested rubella guidelines:

1. Concurrent with initial laboratory studies an HI rubella titer is obtained. If the patient is immune, she is so informed and no further acttion is taken. If she is not immune, it is recommended that she receive rubella vaccine. Adequate contraception for 3 months following vaccination is recommended. Immediate postpartum vaccination may be indicated for certain patients when continuity of care cannot be assured. Rubella vaccination is contraindicated during pregnancy. The choice of timing depends on the patient's motivation for continued medical care.

2. If the patient is exposed to rubella during early pregnancy, the laboratory tests previously described should be carried out. The patient is informed of the result. Further action with regard to interruption of pregnancy is left to the patient after appropriate counseling. (At present, rubella does not constitute a legal reason for interruption of pregnancy in some U.S. states.) If the pregnancy is continued, the pediatrician who will care for the baby should be notified.

3. If the patient is exposed to rubella late in pregnancy, the same procedures are carried out in the laboratory. The diagnosis of a fetal infection with rubella is important to the pediatrician, because the newborn may carry and excrete the virus for some months following birth. The implications of preventive medicine in the nursery are obvious.

4. If rubella vaccine has been given inadvertently to a woman who is in the first trimester of pregnancy, she should be informed of the current status of knowledge of rubella immunization. The work of Severn has shown that rubella vaccine produces optic cup damage in the embryo similar to that of the wild virus, and therefore the vaccine may be significantly teratogenic.

Amnionitis

If the diagnosis of amnionitis is made, the situation should be regarded as very dangerous for both mother and infant. The following steps are suggested:

1. Immediately obtain a smear, gram-stain and culture of the cervical discharge.

2. Institute antibiotic therapy in large doses. One might administer ampicillin, 1 to 2 Gm. every 4-6 hours, intravenously; or penicillin, 20 to 30 million units, with kanamycin, 15 mg./kg. every 24 hours.

3. Obtain blood cultures if the temperature exceeds 100°F.

4. Prompt delivery. If oxytocin stimulation of labor will not effect delivery within 2-6 hours, operative intervention is justified. Low-cervical cesarean section is acceptable if childbearing is to be preserved. Cesarean hysterectomy should be considered in a patient whose condition is deteriorating or perhaps as an alternative to classic cesarean section, which must be considered very dangerous in the face of infection.

Herpes

Generalized herpetic infection of the newborn is a serious, usually fatal illness. It is clear that current modes of therapy for this condition are unsatisfactory; therefore prevention is the key to management. Though not proven beyond doubt, the argument that infection occurs during transit through the birth canal seems logical. The suggested management of the gravida at term and in labor with active herpes progenitalis is cesarean section.

Other Infections

Two other maternal infections of great import in neonatal care are toxoplasmosis and cytomegalic inclusion disease. At present, obstetric knowledge is limited with regard to the prediction of prevention of these newborn problems. It should be remembered that neonate victims of cytomegalic inclusion disease continue to excrete the virus for prolonged periods, as rubella victims do.

TOXEMIA OF PREGNANCY

General guidelines are helpful, but individualization of management is often necessary, particularly if underlying hypertensive disease is the problem, rather than pre-eclampsia or eclampsia.

1. Hospitalization is necessary if two of the three paramount signs of the disorder exist. These are edema, hypertension and proteinuria, and they usually appear in that order. A rough guide to the presence of pathologic edema is a weight gain greater than 5 pounds in 1 week, associated with swelling of the hands or face. A blood pressure exceeding 140/90 or an increase over prepregnancy levels of 30 points systolic or 15 points diastolic is abnormal. The excretion of 500 mg. of protein or more in 24 hours is abnormal.

2. True toxemias of pregnancy are cured only by termination of the pregnancy, not by control of the manifestations of the disease. Therefore, if the fetus is mature, medical or surgical induction of labor by amniotomy is performed.

3. If the condition is mild and the fetus is not mature, bed rest may allow the pregnancy to continue. Diuretics (e.g., chlorothiazide) and sedatives (e.g., barbiturates) are often used. Whether or not these drugs contribute to increased perinatal survival is controversial.

4. If the disease is severe or if convulsions supervene (eclampsia), delivery after stabilization for 12-24 hours is usually the best choice, regardless of fetal maturity. Indications of severe disease are blood pressure in excess of 160/110, oliguria of less than 400 ml./24 hours, excretion of more than 2 Gm. of protein per 24 hours and central nervous system manifestations, such as blurring of vision, severe headache and marked hyperflexia. Initial stabilization is carried out with magnesium sulfate. Ten grams given intramuscularly and followed by 4 Gm. by slow intravenous infusion in 5% dextrose is used; or it may all be given by infusion, the dose being approximately 1 Gm./hour. Overdose results in respiratory depression, so careful monitoring of reflexes and respiratory rate is necessary. Urine output must be monitored, because magnesium is excreted almost entirely in the urine, and oliguria may result in high blood levels. Overdosage can be reversed by slow infusion of 10% calcium gluconate. Newborn depression due to magnesium will be discussed in Chapter 2.

1°85⁷

5. Alarming hypertension may be managed by the infusion of hydralazine in a dose of 20-40 mg./L. of infusate. Only a moderate reduction of the hypertension is sought; e.g., a 10-20% decrease in blood pressure. No attempt is made to achieve normotensive blood pressure levels, because this may result in inadequate perfusion.

DIABETES MELLITUS

For details of the extensive and varied problem of diabetes mellitus the reader is referred to the standard obstetric textbooks. General guidelines currently in use are as follows:

1. Diabetes that is manifest only during pregnancy—"gestational diabetes"— still poses some risk to the fetus and the newborn; therefore these are high-risk pregnancies.

2. Insulin rather than an oral agent is indicated during pregnancy.

3. Every effort should be made to avoid either acidosis or hypoglycemia. Class C, D and E diabetics probably should be hospitalized at 30-32 weeks.

4. Most diabetics are delivered in the 37th week. Efforts to determine fetal maturity (previously outlined) are very important. If conditions are favorable for induction of labor, that is preferable; if not, cesarean section is justified. Whether to deliver before maturity or to permit the pregnancy to go to term is a decision that should be carefully based on the clinical condition to the patient, together with corroborating laboratory evidence, such as serial determinations of urinary estriol (see above).

5. Insulin requirements generally increase as pregnancy progresses. Therefore decreasing requirements may signal trouble.

6. Blood sugar and acetone determinations are more accurate reflections of the patient's status than urinary determinations, because of the variable renal threshold for glucose during pregnancy.

7. A prompt reduction in insulin requirement is common following delivery. A useful guideline is to reduce the insulin dosage by half in the 24 hours following delivery.

BLOOD PROBLEMS

A standard format for the anticipation of fetal and newborn hematologic problems is helpful. Nevertheless, individual variation is often
necessary.

ABO Incompatibility

Although more frequent than Rh incompatibility, this disease in the
perinate is so mild that the only indicated procedure antepartum is to
determine the blood types of the mother and father, in expectation of
possible trouble. We have not felt that amniocentesis is justified for this
problem.

Rh Disease of the Perinate

The literature on this subject is vast. The current protocol can be
summarized as follows:

1. At the initial visit the maternal Rh phenotype is determined. If the
patient is Rh-negative, the father's most probable genotype is determined. Knowing the phenotype of previous children may be helpful.

2. If the patient is not sensitized in the Rh system, she is retested for
anti-D antibody at 28 weeks, 26 weeks and immediately postpartum. If
the baby is Rh-positive, the mother receives Rh (D) immune globulin
within 72 hours postpartum, after proper matching. Two of these products are commercially available at this time: RhoGAM and Gamulin Rh.
When the blood type of the infant or fetus is unknown, as in abortion
patients, the immune globulin is given to Rh-negative women.

3. If the patient is sensitized, the progress of the fetus is
monitored by amniocentesis performed every 2 weeks from about 22 to
24 weeks' gestation. If readily available, placental localization studies
prior to amniotic tap are desirable. The deviation from normal optical
density at $450\,\mu$ on a standard spectrophotometer reflects the severity
of fetal involvement. Our procedure is to vary patient management
according to the zones described by Liley (Fig. 1-1). A numerical value
is obtained from the spectrophotometer (Fig. 1-2). This number is
placed on the graph, at the appropriate week of gestation, each time

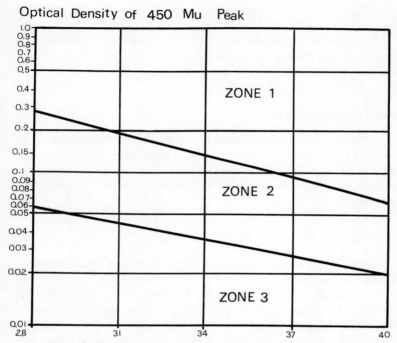

Fig. 1-1.—Liley's zones indicating severity of fetal involvement as reflected by spectrophotometric analysis of amniotic fluid. (From Liley, A. W.: Amniocentesis and Amniography in Hemolytic Disease, in Greenhill, J. P. (ed.): Year Book of Obstetrics and Gynecology, 1964-65 series (Chicago: Year Book Medical Publishers, Inc., 1964) p. 256.

the patient is tapped. If the values are consistently in zone 1, the baby is probably not affected or else is Rh-negative, and no interference is indicated. Generally, if the values are in zone 2 the baby is affected. In most of these cases preterm delivery by induction of labor at fetal maturity is indicated. If the values fall into zone 3, it is anticipated that intrauterine death due to erythroblastosis fetalis is imminent. If the baby is mature enough to survive an extrauterine existence, immediate delivery is carried out; if not, intrauterine transfusion is indicated.

Irregular Antibodies

All patients are screened for antibodies other than those in the ABO

and Rh systems. In our experience, by far the commonest irregular antibodies detected are in the Lewis system. These have caused no serious
perinatal problems, but difficulty in finding compatible blood for maternal transfusions can be anticipated.

Other Blood Problems

Acquired coagulation disorders of pregnancy usually do not affect

Fig. 1-2.—Example of the use of spectrophotometry. Following spectrophotometric examination of amniotic fluid, the deviation at 450 μ is transposed
onto Liley's graph (fig. 1-1). It can be seen that in this patient, at 28 weeks, the
value falls high in zone 2—an indication of probable severe erythroblastosis. If
the value remains in zone 2 on subsequent taps, delivery at the earliest date of
likely extrauterine survival is indicated. (Courtesy of G. William Orr, M.D.,
Associate Professor of Obstetrics, University of Nebraska.)

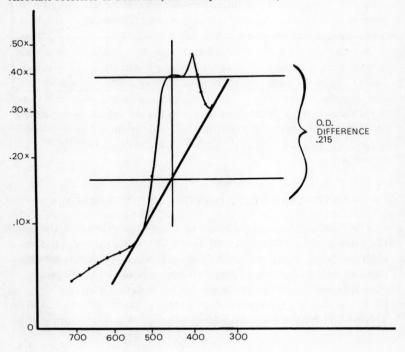

the fetal coagulation system significantly. With regard to hemorrhagic disease of the newborn, the obstetric concept is that transportation of maternally administered vitamin K across the placenta is quite uncertain, and therefore prophylaxis of this problem is more appropriate for the newborn. Maternal thrombocytopenic purpura is worthy of comment, because in the idiopathic variety the neonate often has the passive acquired disease, presumably due to transplacental passage of antibody. These babies should not be subjected to surgical procedures, such as circumcision, because they too may be thrombocytopenic. This can occur even though the mother is in remission as a result of splenectomy: the antiplatelet antibody persists.

Most of the abnormalities of formation of adult hemoglobin, such as sickle-cell disease, are not manifest in the newborn; this is because most of the neonate's hemoglobin is fetal hemoglobin. An exception is homozygous alpha-thalassemia, a condition in which normal fetal hemoglobin cannot be synthesized, and intrauterine or neonatal death due to nonimmunologic erythroblastosis is common. Negro mothers should be routinely screened for sickle-cell disease.

Another common blood disorder in Negroes is glucose-6-phosphate dehydrogenase deficiency. This sex-linked enzyme defect afflicts over 10% of our Negro patients. These patients may develop a hemolytic anemia upon exposure to certain drugs (e.g., sulfas) or chemicals (e.g., naphthalene). If a mother is homozygous for the defect, all her male children will of course have the disorder, and she should be cautioned against exposing the newborn to moth balls and other naphtha products.

ANTENATAL DETECTION OF GENETIC DISORDERS

This subject is beyond the scope of this chapter. However, the primary physician of the pregnant woman should be aware of the fact that by analysis of amniotic fluid and by tissue-culture technics it is possible to make antenatal diagnoses of certain genetic disorders. At the present time, it is possible to determine the sex of the fetus and to detect Down's syndrome, glycogen-storage diseases, enzyme defects and so on. The work of Nadler and others demonstrates the dramatic turn that intrauterine medicine has taken. Most of the sophisticated medical centers offer consultation and genetic counseling on these problems.

AMNIOCENTESIS TECHNIC

The several allusions in this chapter to amniocentesis prompt a brief description of our current technics. Local experience and the literature support the view that amniocentesis, properly undertaken for various reasons, has a value that outweighs the risks. The following indications have been described:

1. Placental localization prior to the tap is desirable, but is not an absolute prerequisite.

2. Amniocentesis is difficult to perform prior to 16 weeks' gestation.

3. The procedure can be performed on outpatients. The abdomen is exposed, prepared and draped as for any other minor outpatient procedure requiring sterility. Sterile gloves and masks are used. The bladder should be empty.

4. A midline tap avoids traumatizing the abdominal wall vessels. Usually, 5 cm. below the umbilicus is the appropriate place of entry; but of course this varies with the size of the uterus.

5. Any standard local anesthetic agent may be used. After anesthesia a 20- or 22-gauge standard spinal needle is used to make a tap. The commercial disposable spinal tray contains most of the necessary equipment.

6. If the tap is bloody or if fluid is not obtained or if the placenta is anterior, an assistant may displace the presenting fetal part out of the pelvis. The tap may then be made just over the symphysis pubis.

7. Ten to 20 ml. of fluid is adequate for most examinations. If genetic studies are to be done, the geneticist should be notified in advance, so that appropriate tissue-culture preparations can be made.

8. The fluid should be collected in a dark bottle, because light destroys bilirubin pigments.

9. Prompt centrifugation is important if the fluid is contaminated with blood or meconium. These substances interfere with spectrophotometric and chemical determinations.

10. If special procedures are to be carried out, it may be appropriate to freeze the fluid in order to maintain accuracy. An example is the de-

termination of the lecithin-sphingomyelin ratio, which must be done promptly, or the fluid must be frozen.

11. Fetal heart tones should be monitored before and after the procedure.

SUGGESTED READINGS

1. Aronson, M.E., and Nelson, P. K.: Fatal air embolism in pregnancy resulting from an unusual sexual act, Obst. & Gynec. 30:127, 1967.
2. Barter, R. H., Hsu, I., and Erkenbeck, R. V.: The prevention of prematurity in multiple pregnancy, Am. J. Obst. & Gynec. 91:787, 1965.
3. Committee on Maternal Nutrition, Food and Nutrition Board, National Research Council: *Maternal Nutrition and the Course of Pregnancy.* (Washington, D.C.: National Academy of Sciences, 1970).
4. Drogemuller, W., Jackson, C., Makowski, E. L., and Battaglia, F. C.: Examination of amniotic fluid as an aid in the assessment of gestational age, Am. J. Obst. & Gynec. 104:424, 1969.
5. Farquhar, J. D.: Results with the Cendehill rubella vaccine in postpartum women, Obst. & Gynec. 35:841, 1970.
6. Gluck, L.: Pulmonary surfactant and neonatal respiratory distress, Hosp. Pract. 6:45, 1971.
7. Gorman, J. G.: Rh immunoglobulin in prevention of hemolytic disease of the newborn child, New York J. Med. 68:1270, 1968.
8. Hon, E. H., and Khazain, A. F.: Observations on fetal heart rate and fetal biochemistry: I. Base deficit, Am. J. Obst. & Gynec. 105:721, 1969.
9. Josey, W. E., Nahmias, A. J., Naib, Z. M., Utley, P. M., McKenzie, W. J., and Coleman, M. T.: Genital herpes simplex infection in the female, Am. J. Obst. & Gynec. 107:807, 1970.
10. Klopper, A.: Assessment of fetoplacental function by hormone assay, Am. J. Obst. & Gynec. 107:807, 1970.
11. Kyle, G. C.: Diabetes in pregnancy, Ann. Int. Med. 59 (Suppl. 31): 1, 1963.
12. Landesman, R., Wilson, F., and Zlatnik, F.: Myometrial relaxant properties of isoxsuprine and two methanesulforamide derivatives, Obst. & Gynec. 28:775, 1966.
13. Larson, A. L., Engstrom, A. W.: The determination of estrogen and progesterone metabolites in urine in pregnancy by gas chromatography, Am. J. Clin. Path. 46:352, 1966.

14. Liley, A. W.: Amniocentesis and Amniography in Hemolytic Disease, in *Year Book of Obstetrics and Gynecology,* 1964-65 Series (Chicago: Year Book Medical Publishers, 1964), p. 256.
15. Lopez, R., and Cooperman, J. M.: Glucose-6-phosphate dehydrogenase deficiency and hyperbilirubinemia in the newborn, Am. J. Dis. Child. 122:66, 1971.
16. McDonald, I. A.: Incompetent cervix as a cause of recurrent abortion, J. Obst. & Gynaec. Brit. Commonwealth 70:105, 1963.
17. Messer, R. H.: Heat stable alkaline phosphatase as an index of placental function, Am. J. Obst. & Gynec. 98:459, 1967.
18. Meyer, H. M., and Parkman, P. D.: Rubella vaccination, J.A.M.A., 215:613, 1971.
19. Nadler, H. L.: Indications for Amniocentesis in the Early Prenatal Detection of Genetic Disorders, in Bergsma, D. (ed.): *Symposium on Intrauterine Diagnosis,* National Foundation, Birth Defects, Orig. Art. Ser. 7:(5) April, 1971.
20. Naeye, R. L.: Malnutrition: probable cause of fetal growth retardation, Arch. Path. 79:284, 1965.
21. O'Sullivan, J. B., Charles, D., and Dandrow, R. V.: Treatment of verified prediabetics in pregnancy, J. Reproductive Med. 7:21, 1971.
22. Pritchard, J. A.: The use of the magnesium ion in the management of eclamptogenic toxemias, Surg., Gynec. & Obst. 100:131, 1955.
23. Rausen, A. R., Seki, M., and Strauss, L.: Twin transfusion syndrome, a review of 19 cases studied at one institution, J. Pediat. 66:613, 1965.
24. Reid, D. E.: Diabetes mellitus in pregnancy, Internat. J. Gynec. & Obst. 9:1, 1971.
25. Rubella virus vaccine, recommendations of the Advisory Committee of Immunization Practices, U.S.P.H.S., Ann. Int. Med. 73:779, 1970.
26. Sharma, S. D., and Trussell, R. R.: The value of amniotic fluid examination in assessment of fetal maturity, J. Obst. & Gynaec. Brit. Commonwealth 77:215, 1970.
27. Stone, S. R., and Pritchard, J. A.: Effect of maternally administered magnesium sulfate on the neonate, Obst. & Gynec. 35:574, 1970.
28. Webb, G. A.: Maternal death associated with premature rupture of the membranes, Am. J. Obst. & Gynec. 98:594, 1967.
29. Yerushalmy, J.: The low-birthweight baby, Hosp. Pract. 3:62, 1968.

CHAPTER 2

Maternal Factors and General Care of the Newborn

G. VAN LEEUWEN, M.D.

The first chapter of this book could itself have been developed into a textbook. In the present chapter, certain high spots will be mentioned from the standpoint of the effect various maternal factors have on the unborn infant. Routine general care of normal newborn infants also will be discussed, as well as some variations from the normal.

Any situation adversely affecting a pregnant woman is likely to, or at least may, adversely affect the unborn infant. Very little is known about the cause of birth defects, but it is probable that environment, drugs ingested and illnesses suffered by the mother are significantly involved in the production of defective children. Most is known about infection; something is known about drugs; little is known about other factors. As for the use of drugs: one can reprimand women who are demonstrably pregnant, but it is much more difficult to reprimand them when pregnancy is only potential or is not yet fully obvious.

PRENATAL CARE

The importance of adequate prenatal care is recognized by all practitioners of obstetrics and newborn medicine, although absolute evidence and specific data are lacking. One must begin with the concept that the physical, mental and emotional patterns of the future child are present in each parent prior to the time of conception but that the extent to which they involve the infant are almost totally unknown. A wide range of antenatal influences may be responsible for an abnormal infant. Broadly, these influences can be grouped into three categories: (1) the effect of abnormal genetic structure, (2) the effect of chromosomal changes and (3) the effect of abnormal intrauterine influence. Some examples are isoimmunization and hemolytic disease of the presence of galactosemia and phenylketonuria. The list of and sex-chromosome abnormalities continues to grow. Intrauterine tors might include malnutrition, radiation and infection.

It has become apparent that regular prenatal visits to the physician have significantly reduced both maternal and infant mortality.

Perinatal factors are of equal significance, and these will be referred to intermittently throughout this chapter. It is obvious that all infants should be delivered by a thoroughly competent and well-trained person, whether this be a physician or a physician's assistant. The choice of anesthesia, sedation and method of delivery will significantly affect the offspring. The first day of life (which is included in the perinatal period) is the most critical in one's entire life. Disorders in this time period will be discussed later.

NUTRITION

The significance of poor nutrition in the pregnant woman is not thoroughly understood. Clear-cut studies in certain animal species suggest that nutritional deprivation toward the end of gestation significantly decreases the size of the offspring. The physical maturation of the human fetus, however, seems to be much less vulnerable to maternal undernourishment. Studies done during periods of extreme poverty in Japan and the Netherlands showed only a slight decrease in birthweight (7-10%) in the presence of severe nutritional shortage in the pregnant female. A number of studies have suggested that there may be permanent damage to the brain if nutritional restriction is imposed at a time when the brain is undergoing its period of most rapid growth. (In the human, of course, this occurs during the last few months of normal gestation, as well as in the early life of the infant.) Other studies have suggested that human brain development is independent of unfavorable gestational circumstances which may affect physical growth. Altogether, at the present time one cannot make a definitive statement about the effect of nutrition on the infant.

ILLNESSES OF THE MOTHER WHICH AFFECT THE BABY

Although any illness in the mother may adversely affect the infant, there are three about which there is the greatest concern and of which medical science has the greatest degree of understanding. These are diabetes, toxemia and infection during pregnancy—particularly infection with viruses.

Diabetes

Until the discovery of insulin, pregnancy carried to completion was a rare occurrence in diabetic women. As the care of the diabetic has improved, so has success in pregnancy: probably 65-70% of all conceptions in diabetic mothers now result in live births. But this is to say that some 35% of all such conceptions still end in death. The majority of these are intrauterine early and late abortions; a smaller portion are neonatal deaths. During the past several years the significant decrease in mortality in this category has been through decrease in intrauterine deaths at the termination of pregnancy. Placental-function tests—particularly the urinary test of estriol output in the mother—have made it possible to determine more accurately the correct time at which an infant should be delivered.

The infant of the diabetic mother will be discussed in a later chapter in some detail. A host of problems occur in these infants. The most common causes of death are respiratory distress syndrome, infection and congenital malformations. These infants are more likely to suffer from hyperbilirubinemia, hypoglycemia and hypocalcemic tetany. However, cumulative evidence does indicate that, irrespective of the severity of the mother's diabetes, those mothers who are well controlled by a diabetic team have the greatest likelihood of producing reasonably healthy infants.

Toxemia of Pregnancy

Infants born to mothers who have toxemia have approximately a 20% mortality rate—which is comparable to the death rate in infants born prior to 36 weeks' gestation. Death usually occurs very early in the neonatal period and is secondary to depression of the infant. How much of this is due to the disease process and how much is due to the antihypertensive drugs given to the mother is not clear.

Infants of toxemic mothers are susceptible to most of the disorders common to infants born before the 36th week; these include respiratory distress syndrome, septicemia and hypoglycemia. One particular affliction—hypermagnesemia—has been described only recently. In mothers who have received magnesium sulfate as an antihypertensive agent, an unpredictable amount of the drug crosses the placenta. There are increasing reports of infants born with hypermagnesemia sufficient to produce clinical symptoms including, in some instances, respiratory paralysis. Serum magnesium levels should be obtained in all newborns of toxemic mothers who have received magnesium sulfate. If the level is sufficiently high to produce respiratory depression—often the only physical sign, along with absence of reflexes—an exchange transfusion should promptly be performed. The recovery may be dramatic; but lack of treatment is very likely to to fatal.

Infection

Any infection in the mother is potentially damaging to the fetus. Infection during the first trimester, particularly with viruses, may give rise to birth defects. Infection in the last trimester of pregnancy may produce an infant who is infected at birth. Last-trimester infections, too, are primarily caused by viruses; but there are instances of congenital bacterial infections which were apparently present in spite of intact amniotic membranes. The management of infants born to mothers who are or have been infected is described in the Chapter 8.

RECOGNIZING THE RISK INFANT

There are a number of conditions in which it is apparent that the infant is at risk. These are:

1. Low birthweight.
2. Low birthweight for gestational age.
3. Maternal diabetes.
4. Maternal toxemia.

5. Blood incompatibility.
6. Congenital malformation.
7. Any form of complicated pregnancy, labor or delivery, including placental insufficiency.

Careful prenatal history will indicate the likelihood of a risk infant 60% of the time. Disease in the mother during or before pregnancy assists in the recognition. Inadequate intrauterine growth suggests that the pregnancy is becoming risky. The problems during labor and at birth readily indicate risk babies.

The illnesses encountered in risk infants are standard and are all discussed in various chapters of this book. They are, primarily, the following seven:

1. Infection.
2. Hyaline membrane syndrome.
3. Hypoglycemia and hypocalcemia.
4. Hyperbilirubinemia.
5. Anoxia and apnea.
6. Metabolic and respiratory acidosis.
7. Congenital malformation.

ESTIMATION OF GESTATIONAL AGE

Much has been written in recent years about the importance of recognizing the gestational age of the newborn infant rather than simply declaring him "mature" or "premature." Three charts are reproduced here to assist the reader in making his own estimation of gestational age. Table 2-1 and Figures 2-1 and 2-2—the Colorado Intrauterine Growth Charts—when plotted against gestational age provide an excellent prognostic indicator of the outcome for a particular infant. This benefits the parents and contributes to the peace of mind of the physician; furthermore, one can predict early whether the infant should be transferred to a newborn intensive-care unit or treated as a normal infant.

TRANSITIONAL NURSERY

Most hospital nurseries are designed to care for the 80%-90% of infants who are normal and have no problems during the neonatal period. In recent years there has been a greater tendency to place highly skilled personnel in high-risk nurseries, which now are filled with electronic equipment. Such a nursery may indeed be called an intensive-care unit.

Except under optimal situations in hospitals where a full-time practitioner of newborn medicine is present, most newborn infants are not examined within the first hour of life. More often than not they are examined the following morning or at a convenient time for the physician after his office hours and emergencies are over. The newborn infant, however, should be considered a recovering patient, especially when the mother has received analgesia and anesthesia during labor and delivery. Therefore, our institution has a special nursery to which the newborn are admitted for a minium of 24 hours following delivery.

The transitional-care nursery should primarily be equipped with some form of infant warmer, so that adequate body temperature may be maintained without having to cover or wrap up the infant. Monitoring equipment is mandatory. We believe that two or three of the following should be constantly monitored: heart rate, respiratory rate and body temperature. If at any time during the 24-hour period he is in the transitional-care nursery the infant appears to be ill, he is immediately transferred to the high-risk nursery.

A highly skilled nurse should be in attendance in the transitional nursery. It is not particularly desirable that these nurses bathe the infants and do the other routine admitting procedures, but it is imperative that they be there to recognize the infant who is not doing well. In our institution these nurses have been trained to perform the congenital-anomaly survey and to promptly recognize respiratory distress, cyanosis, seizures and other deviations from normal.

The immature infant reacts to birth in a slower fashion than the term infant. His thermoregulatory mechanism is less well established, he is more likely to develop respiratory distress, and apnea spells are more common. The infant whose birthweight is extremely low is immediately admitted to the high-risk nursery. The borderline small-for-date infant is admitted to the transitional nursery, inasmuch as he may be totally normal at 12-24 hours of age. Hypoglycemia is often encountered in risk infants during the first 24 hours.

Table 2-1. CLINICAL ASSESSMENT OF GESTATIONAL AGE IN THE NEWBORN INFANT*

External Sign	Score:** 0	1	2	3	4
Edema	Obvious edema of hands and feet; pitting over tibia	No obvious edema of hands and feet; pitting over tibia	No edema		
Skin texture	Very thin, gelatinous	Thin and smooth	Smooth: medium thickness, rash or superficial peeling	Slight thickening; superficial cracking and peeling, especially of hands and feet	Thick and parchment-like; superficial or deep cracking
Skin color	Dark red	Uniformly pink	Pale pink; variable over body	Pale; only pink over ears, lips, palms, or soles	
Skin opacity (trunk)	Numerous veins and venules clearly seen, especially over abdomen	Veins and tributaries seen	A few large vessels clearly seen over abdomen	A few large vessels seen indistinctly over abdomen	No blood vessels seen
Lanugo (over back)	No lanugo	Abundant; long and thick over whole back	Hair thinning, especially over lower back	Small amount of lanugo and bald areas	At least half of back devoid of lanugo
Plantar creases	No skin creases	Faint red marks over anterior half of sole	Definite red marks over anterior half; indentations over anterior third	Indentations over anterior third	Definite deep indentations over anterior third

Nipple formation	Nipple barely visible; no areola	Nipple well defined; areola smooth and flat; diameter 0.75 cm.	Areola stippled, edge not raised; diameter 0.75 cm.	Areola stippled, edge raised; diameter 0.75 cm.
Breast size	No breast tissue palpable	Breast tissue on one or both sides; diameter 0.5 cm.	Breast tissue on both sides; one or both 0.5-1.0 cm.	Breast tissue on both sides; one or both 1.0 cm.
Ear form	Pinna flat and shapeless; little or no curving of edge	Incurving of part of edge of pinna	Partial incurving of whole of upper pinna	Well-defined incurving of whole of upper pinna
Ear firmness	Pinna soft, easily folded; no recoil	Pinna soft, easily folded; slow recoil	Cartilage to edge of pinna but soft in places; ready recoil	Pinna firm, cartilage to edge; instant recoil
Genitals Male	Neither testis in scrotum	At least one testis high in scrotum	At least one testis right down	
Female (with hips half abducted)	Labia majora widely separated, labia minora protruding	Labia majora almost cover labia minora	Labia majora completely cover labia minora	

* Adapted from Farr *et al.*, Developmental Med. & Child Neurol. 8:507, 1966. See also J. Pediat. 77:1, 1970.
** If score differs on two sides, take the mean.

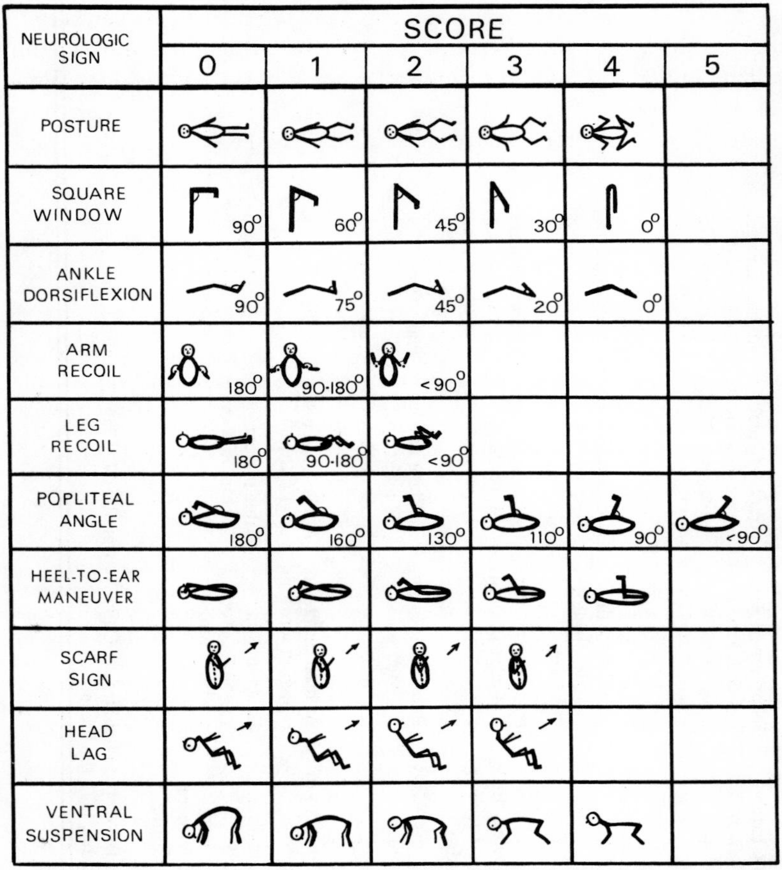

NEUROLOGIC SIGN	SCORE					
	0	1	2	3	4	5
POSTURE						
SQUARE WINDOW	90°	60°	45°	30°	0°	
ANKLE DORSIFLEXION	90°	75°	45°	20°	0°	
ARM RECOIL	180°	90-180°	<90°			
LEG RECOIL	180°	90-180°	<90°			
POPLITEAL ANGLE	180°	160°	130°	110°	90°	<90°
HEEL-TO-EAR MANEUVER						
SCARF SIGN						
HEAD LAG						
VENTRAL SUSPENSION						

Fig. 2-1.—Scoring system for neurologic criteria; from Dubowitz, L. M. S., Dubowitz, V., and Goldberg, C.: Clinical assessment of gestational age in the newborn infant, J. Pediat. 77:1, 1970. If the score differs on the two sides, take the mean. The following are notes, from the same source, on technics of assessment:

Posture. Observed with infant quiet and in supine position. Score O: arms and legs extended; 1: beginning of flexion of hips and knees, arms extended; 2: stronger flexion of legs, arms extended; 3: arms slightly flexed, legs flexed and abducted; 4: full flexion of arms and legs.

Square window. The hand is flexed on the forearm between the thumb and index finger of the examiner. Enough pressure is applied to get as full a flexion as possible, and the angle between the hypothenar eminence and the ventral aspect of the forearm is measured and graded according to diagram. (Care is taken not to rotate the infant's wrist while doing this maneuver.)

All anesthetic and analgesic agents potentially depress the newborn infant. This is particularly true of narcotics. The recent use of magnesium sulfate in the treatment of toxemia of pregnancy has resulted in respiratory depression and lethargy in the newborn. All infants depressed by maternal medication may have apnea spells, may be extremely lethargic, and are likely to vomit and aspirate.

Ankle dorsiflexion. The foot is dorsiflexed onto the anterior aspect of the leg, with the examiner's thumb on the sole of the foot and other fingers behind the leg. Enough pressure is applied to get as full flexion as possible, and the angle between the dorsum of the foot and the anterior aspect of the leg is measured.

Arm recoil. With the infant in the supine position the forearms are first flexed for 5 seconds, then fully extended by pulling on the hands, and then released. The sign is fully positive if the arms return briskly to full flexion (score 2). If the arms return to incomplete flexion or the response is sluggish, it is graded as score 1. If they remain extended or are only followed by random movements the score is 0.

Leg recoil. With the infant supine, the hips and knees are fully flexed for 5 seconds, then extended by traction on the feet and released. A maximal response is one of full flexion of the hips and knees (score 2). A partial flexion scores 1, and minimal or no movement scores 0.

Popliteal angle. With the infant supine and his pelvis flat on the examining couch, the thigh is held in the knee-chest position by the examiner's left index finger and thumb supporting the knee. The leg is then extended by gentle pressure from the examiner's right index finger behind the ankle, and the popliteal angle is measured.

Heel-to-ear maneuver. With the baby supine, draw the baby's foot as near to the head as it will go without forcing it. Observe the distance between the foot and the head as well as the degree of extension at the knee. Grade according to diagram. Note that the knee is left free and may draw down alongside the abdomen.

Scarf sign. With the baby supine, take the infant's hand and try to put it around the neck and as far posteriorly as possible around the opposite shoulder. Assist this maneuver by lifting the elbow across the body. See how far the elbow will go across and grade according to illustrations. Score 0: elbow reaches opposite axillary line; 1: elbow between midline and opposite axillary line; 2: elbow reaches midline; 3: elbow will not reach midline.

Head lag. With the baby lying supine, grasp the hands (or the arms if a very small infant) and pull him slowly towards the sitting position. Observe the position of the head in relation to the trunk and grade accordingly. In a small infant the head may initially be supported by one hand. Score 0: complete lag; 1: partial head control; 2: able to maintain head in line with body; 3: brings head anterior to body.

Ventral suspension. The infant is suspended in the prone position, with examiner's hand under the infant's chest (one hand in a small infant, two in a large infant). Observe the degree of extension of the back and the amount of flexion of the arms and legs. Also note the relation of the head to the trunk. Grade according to diagram.

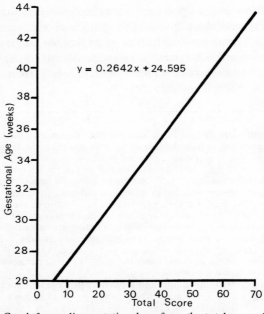

Fig. 2-2.—Graph for reading gestational age from the total score obtained by the use of Fig. 2-1. (Same source.)

All babies with Apgar scores of 7 or less are most carefully observed for at least 24 hours. They are admitted to the high-risk nursery directly or later on. Apnea spells are more common in these infants; so are seizures.

In order to prevent the very common occurrence of hypoglycemia in risk infants, all of our infants are fed by 12 hours of age, and the smaller infants are fed by 6 hours of age. The infant with the low Apgar score presents a particular problem in this regard. We believe it is important that the first one or two feedings be administered by a skilled person, because these are the only feedings with which difficulty is usually encountered. During this time the nurse will also recognize the infant who has a poor sucking reflex or an exaggerated gag reflex. The nurses check infants for hypoglycemia frequently with Dextrostix.

Our nurses are all carefully instructed in the congenital-anomaly appraisal and perform this within the first hour of life. (The appraisal is described in Chapter 4.) A peripheral hematocrit is done by the nurse on all infants, before age 1 hour. In all infants in whom difficulty is anticipated (e.g., by reason of difficult labor or pregnancy) Dextrostix is done by the nurse as often as she thinks necessary, and hypoglycemia of less than 45 mg./100 ml. is immediately reported to the house physician.

To some people these procedures may seem expensive and unnecessary, for only 10% of infants develop problems. Yet it is in this 10% that many deaths occur, that many congenital malformations occur, and that much mental retardation is seen as an ultimate sequela. For this reason we believe that a transitional nursery for all newborns is as important as a high-risk nursery for the patently sick newborn. The sick newborn can, in small community hospitals, be transferred to the pediatric floor; although this may not be desirable, it does provide good care. The normal newborn needs no special care. However, the infant with an unsuspected abnormality may become critically ill, may suffer brain damage or may even die in the normal-newborn nursery, where he is wrapped up, unexposed, and often not looked at for 2 or 3 hours. The cost of equipment is minimal, depending upon the size of the delivery service. Three to five infant warmers and three to five monitors cost a total of about $5,000. This is far less than the cost of treating, for life, even one patient institutionalized for mental retardation.

In summary: we consider newborns to be postoperative recovering patients until they have totally recovered from the effects of labor and delivery. Neonatal difficulties usually have their onset in the first few hours of life; and the course of all infants from the moment of birth is unpredictable. For these reasons we believe skilled nursing personnel, well trained in the problems of the newborn and capable of recognizing deviations form normal, should be primarily responsible for all newborn infants during the first 24 hours of life.

FEEDING

The practice of withholding calories and water from the newborn infant for 48-72 hours until diuresis has occurred and edema has disappeared has been replaced by the practice of early feeding. The time of first feeding is probably of very little importance to the normal, term infant.

We institute feedings at 6-12 hours of age, primarily so that the infant will have taken sufficient milk by the time of discharge, so that the Guthrie test for phenylketonuria will be accurate. Similarly, the practice of giving several water feedings prior to milk feedings has been replaced by a single sterile-water feeding to acquaint the infant with what he is expected to do. If he tolerates a single water feeding satisfactorily, there is no good reason to repeat water. A full-strength artificial formula is introduced at 16 hours of age, as desired. In infants taking human milk, small amounts of water are given every 4 hours after the baby has been to the breast, to keep the infant reasonably quiet. On about the second day, when arrival of breast milk is to be expected, water is withheld from the infant so that the breasts are properly stimulated.

Feeding of the small or risk infant should be done in the first 3-6 hours of life. The primary reason for this is not to provide water to the infant but to provide calories, and particularly glucose. Most hypoglycemia of the low-birthweight infant and the infant of a toxemic mother can be prevented by early feeding. Some hypoglycemia of the infant of a diabetic mother can be modified and prevented in the same manner. In infants who weigh 1,200-2,500 Gm., fluids by nipple or gavage are initiated at 3 hours of age in an attempt to prevent hypoglycemia, as well as acidosis. If the infant weighs less than 1,200 Gm., parenteral fluids are immediately instituted. This is done for two reasons: (1) provide glucose and (2) to have a ready vehicle for the administration of medication and for obtaining of blood gas studies, should the infant develop distress. At least half the infants weighing less than 1,200 Gm. develop some difficulty, so that this procedure is strongly justified. The healthy small infant is given a dilute milk formula after one or two water feedings and then progresses to a full-strength formula, as tolerated. The distressed infant or the infant who weighs less than 1,200 Gm. is given oral feedings as soon as he tolerates them, and parenteral fluids are discontinued when the full level of 150 ml./kg. is reached. All infants should, by 72 hours, be receiving 150 ml./kg. of fluids, and by the fifth day of life they should all be receiving a total caloric intake compatible with growth. This caloric requirement is approximately 100 cal./kg. in the term infant and 120 cal./kg. in the low-birthweight infant. Both the morbidity and the mortality of low-birthweight infants have been reduced when the only known variable factor introduced was feeding at less than 6 hours of age.

The only possible objection to early feeding is the likelihood of aspiration. Again, if the infant is in a transitional nursery or in a high-risk unit the likelihood of aspiration is minimized. Infants in respiratory distress who must lie on their backs with umbilical catheters in place should not be fed; this must wait until they can be placed in a lateral position or on the abdomen.

EYE AND CORD CARE

Eye

Some form of prophylactic therapy to prevent gonorrheal ophthalmia is required in all U.S. states. The laws vary from state to state, but some agent that is lethal to the gonorrheal organism must be instilled shortly after birth. After attempting many different forms of eye prophylaxis, we have returned to, and have been most satisfied with, the instillation of a 2% silver nitrate solution, two drops in each eye at the time of birth. When the eyes are properly irrigated, 15 seconds later, chemical conjunctivitis is minimal and the antibacterial effect is near 100%.

Nevertheless, we continue to encounter patients with gonorrheal ophthalmia. These patients present at 5 to 7 days of age in the emergency room, and they are of the reinfection type. This form of the disease is increasing in frequency. We continue to treat it systemically with large doses of penicillin and with aqueous penicillin solution irrigation of the eyes every 20-30 minutes until the infection regresses.

Cord

The care of the cord after birth is of little significance if the cord is clamped as close to the skin as possible. Even in Rh-sensitized infants we prefer the very close clamping and dry cord, not only to minimize the risk of infection but also because at the time of insertion of the umbilical catheter the cord is cut this close anyhow. The wide plastic clamp is the most desirable device for clamping the cord, because there is less likelihood that the cord will be cut than with a metal clamp or umbilical tape. To prevent damage to the umbilical structures the cord clamp should be at right angles to the infant's longitudinal axis. Whether the cord is washed with peroxide or alcohol or is not washed at all is of no importance, we believe.

CIRCUMCISION

Because circumcision of the male in this country has become essentially routine, we hesitate to devote space to a discussion of it. We have always been opposed to routine circumcision except when it is indicated for religious reasons. We are aware that the arguments for circumcision are somewhat impressive with respect to the increased incidence of malignancy of the cervix and of the penis, as well as the fact that cleanliness is easier without the foreskin being present. On the other hand, we believe that the smegma that accumulates beneath the foreskin is the carcinogenic agent, not the foreskin itself. We have talked with a number of men who were circumcised as adults; they said that sexual intercourse is less satisfying to them than it had been before circumcision. Admittedly, none of them had discontinued the practice because of lack of enjoyment.

We have also seen, however, a number of infants with significant hypospadias who were circumcised before the hypospadias was recognized. This most often occurs when circumcision is done at the time of delivery, in the delivery room. The foreskin is a highly sensitive, highly vascular tissue which can be used as a skin graft in a number of other parts of the body where sensitive skin is desirable. For this reason we think it should be preserved. It is particularly useful in reconstructive surgery of the external genitalia. Needless to say, genital injuries are increasingly common, with the high incidence of motorcycle accidents. On the rare occasion when parents have rejected circumcision, we have done nothing until the child is 1 year old, and then we have instructed the mother as to retraction of the foreskin and proper cleaning. This is a painless procedure after the initial adhesions are broken. If the mother teaches the child to do this for himself, when he becomes older, we believe circumcision is unwarranted.

In spite of these arguments, however, practically all of our patients, like those in other institutions, are circumcised on the third or fourth day of life. We would respectfully insist that, if circumcision continues to be a routine procedure, our obstetric colleagues should at least tell the mother why they think it should be done. We have been impressed by a study conducted by a medical student a number of years ago, in which 100 mothers were queried as to why they had their sons circumcised. Many gave the usual reasons, but some said they had it done because the mother-in-law insisted or because they thought it was required by state law or because they thought "it looked better."

VITAMIN K

It is now generally agreed that the administration of phytonadione (AquaMephyton), or vitamin K, to prevent hemorrhagic disease of the newborn is indicated in all newborn infants. The complications arising from the administration of either 1 mg. intramuscularly or 2 mg. orally are essentially zero, and hemorrhagic disease (or, at least, the variety due to prothrombin deficiency) has almost been eliminated since this procedure was introduced. We are satisfied with either route of administration and find no difference in the incidence of hemorrhage, whether the drug is given orally or intramuscularly.

VARIATIONS FROM NORMAL

Variations from normal in the newborn infant are so common that a textbook might be devoted entirely to this subject. We will simply list here, by anatomic area, those which seem to present the greatest difficulty and confusion to pediatric house officers and students.

The Head

Overriding of the sutures and a small anterior fontanel may indicate microcephaly or may be within normal limits. If the condition is merely related to the small size of the birth canal and to difficulties of delivery, the suture overriding usually disappears by the third or fourth day of life. We do not ordinarily become concerned until that time, unless the head is decidedly small by comparison with the size of the body.

Variation of the ears has little significance unless the ears are low-set. When the helix of the ear is lower than the lateral epicanthus of the eye, the ears are indeed low-set and the infant should be investigated for chromosomal defects and for renal abnormalities.

Hemangiomas of the face and neck are very common, and nearly all of them disappear without treatment; thus no treatment should be suggested until the 18th month of age.

Tongue-tie is a term best forgotten. We now entirely reject the practice of clipping the frenulum in the neonatal period. Incidences of severe hemorrhage have occurred when this has been done.

Occasionally the small size of the mandible gives rise to concern. Unless it is accompanied by cleft palate and glossoptosis (Pierre-Robin syndrome), a small mandible has no significance.

Chest

A significant number of infants have an entity which, for lack of a better term and better understanding, is called transient respiratory distress of the newborn. This is characterized by an expiratory grunt in the first hour of life, without cyanosis and without much discomfort on the part of the infant. The grunt usually disappears without therapy; therefore we do not make the diagnosis of respiratory distress syndrome in first hour of life unless the infant becomes progressively worse.

Systolic heart murmur, often of grade 2 to 4, is frequently heard in the neonatal period. The murmur probably is a reflection of changing hemodynamics and has little significance unless accompanied by other signs of heart disease. It is important to remember that the neonate with severe cyanotic congenital heart disease usually does not have a murmur, because valvular and septal defects are not usually a part of the kind of heart disorder which causes trouble in the neonatal period.

Abdomen

Palpation of the liver, spleen and lower poles of both kidneys is entirely within normal limits in most newborns. Redundancy of the skin of the umbilicus and the presence of a small hernia is also considered to be a minor variation from normal. Most of these hernias rapidly disappear. Undescended testicles are common, but they can often be palpated in the inguinal canal. The clitoris is fairly prominent in many newborns, particularly in the smaller ones. Vaginal adhesions are common; they can be easily lysed with any blunt instrument. Vaginal tags are extremely common and have no clinical significance.

Extremities

Uneven size of the toes, webbed toes, and various forms of eversion and inversion of the foot are all within normal limits provided the malposition can be overcorrected manually. If this cannot be done, there is probably a defect of bone. Abnormalities of the upper extremity are less common.

Skin

Toxic erythema of the newborn is probably not an illness. It occurs in about one of every three infants. It is often confused with pyoderma, and occasionally these infants are isolated and treated with antibacterial agents. Simple but careful examination reveals a yellow vesicular lesion on a red base, which suggests the diagnosis, and the fleeting nature of the condition confirms the diagnosis. Should any doubt remain, a simple Wright stain of the material in the vesicle will demonstrate that the majority of the cells are eosinophilic leukocytes rather than polymorphonuclear leukocytes. Other skin conditions, such as excessive desquamation of the skin, are also within normal limits.

THE SMALL-FOR-DATE INFANT

The small-for-date infant remains a perplexing problem. Unless the gestational age is known, the infant will be called premature, although he may indeed be a term infant. It is wise to remember that (1) not all babies born prematurely need be treated as such—which reduces anxiety and expense; and (2) many problems of the newborn are related to their maturity, not to their size. An excellent review of the small-for-date infant was presented in the February 1970 issue of *Pediatric Clinics of North America.* The entire concept of the small-for-date baby and how the differentiating terms arise are graphically illustrated in Figure 2-3. As the figure makes clear, the small-for-date infant may be postmature, mature, premature or even immature. He may at birth simply be the product of dysmaturity, he may be a dwarf or he may be a normal small child.

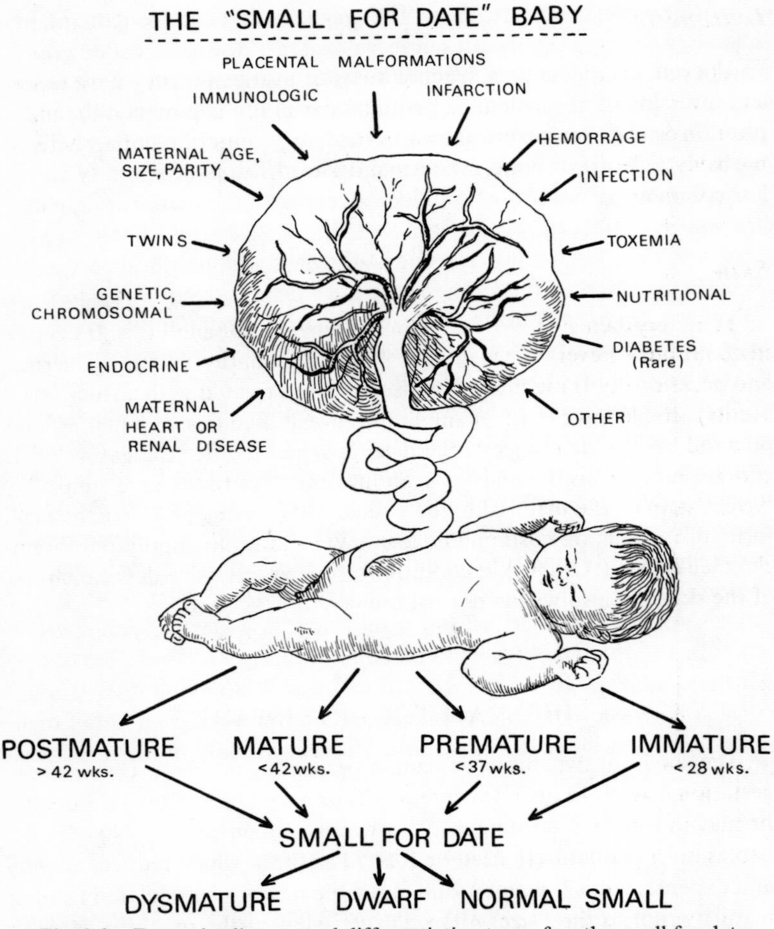

THE "SMALL FOR DATE" BABY

Fig. 2-3.—Events leading to, and differentiating terms for, the small-for-date baby. (From Andrews, B. F.: Symposium, on the small-for-date infant, Pediat. Clin. North America 17:2, 1970; reproduced by permission of the author.)

If one has estimated the gestational age (by the method described earlier in this chapter), one can decide whether the infant is small for the date of gestation. Aside from constitutional factors, the most likely explanation of a small-for-date infant is disease in the mother or a placental malformation or insufficiency. The diagnosis of small-for-date infant calls attention to a significant number of infants, formerly called premature babies, and to their specific series of problems. They have represented a significant segment of perinatal morbidity and mortality, and quite likely they have contributed to the large group of children with cerebral palsy, mental retardation and other major defects.

An impressive number of problems occur with the small-for-date infant who is dysmature. Aside from looking very thin, he is likely to have a dry wrinkled skin, yellow staining of the nails and umbilical cord and respiratory distress at birth. The respiratory distress is not related to hyaline membrane syndrome; instead, it usually is amnionitis. Treatment is very unsatisfactory, but it is best aimed at proper oxygenation and the prevention of bacterial superinfection.

These babies appear to be unusually alert: they cry when touched, and they seem constantly to be staring at their surroundings. They have a high incidence of polycythemia and of refractory hypoglycemia, which is often totally unresponsive to glucose given parenterally and is only alleviated by phlebotomy. There is also a high incidence of hyperuricemia. Dysmature infants tend to have abnormal neurologic signs, including seizures.

The symptoms are best treated specifically; however, only the polycythemia and the hypoglycemia can be satisfactorily treated. It is likely that these infants have been anoxic in utero, and supplying sufficient oxygen simply prevents further damage. These infants have a rather high morbidity but a fairly low mortality. The recognizably dysmature infant occurs in about 2% of pregnancies.

THE HEALTHY PRETERM INFANT

Many babies, but particularly those weighing over 1,500 Gm., who are born before 38 weeks' gestation require very little in the way of special care. They are fed early but in other respects are managed in much the same way as normal, term infants. The earlier their gestational age, the more likely they are to experience the difficulties common to these infants and the more intently they must be observed.

We are not compulsive about keeping all of these infants in the hospital until they reach a weight of 2,500 Gm. We are willing to send them home to competent parents when they have demonstrated their ability to gain weight, maintain their body temperature and feed properly. With all our infants, including those who are ill, we encourage the parents to come to the hospital, to participate in their child's care and to feed him. This reduces the emotional deprivation which takes place—certainly in the mother and quite likely in the infant.

SUGGESTED READINGS

1. Andrews, B. F., Lorchirachoonkul, V., and Shott, R. J.: Small-for-date-babies, Pediat. Clin. North America 17:185, 1970.
2. Bloxsom, A.: The function of a recovery nursery in a large maternity hospital, J. Pediat. 38:618, 1951.
3. Brady, J., and Williams, H.: Magnesium intoxication in a premature infant, Pediatrics 40:100, 1967.
4. Cornblath, M., Joassin, G., Weisskopf, B., and Swiatek, K. R.: Hypoglycemia in the newborn, Pediat. Clin. North America 13:905, 1966.
5. Craig, W. S.: Congenital Anomalies, in *Care of the Newly Born Infant* (Baltimore: The Williams & Wilkins Co., 1969).
6. Craig, W. S.: Minor Departures from Normal, in *Care of the Newly Born Infant* (Baltimore: The Williams & Wilkins Co., 1969).
7. Desmond, M. M., Randolph, A. J., and Phitaksphraiwan, P.: The transitional care nursery. A mechanism for preventive medicine in the newborn, Pediat. Clin. North America 13:651, 1966.
8. Desmond, M. M., *et al.:* The clinical behavior of the newly born. I. The term baby, J. Pediat. 62:307, 1963.
9. Dobbing, J.: Vulnerable Periods in Developing Brain, in *Applied Neuro-Chemistry* (Oxford: Blackwell, 1968).
10. Gruenwald, P.: The fetus in prolonged pregnancy, Am. J.Obst. & Gynec. 89:504, 1964.
11. Gruenwald, P.: Chronic fetal distress and placental insufficiency, Biologia Neonatorum 5:215, 1963.
12. Hughes, W. T.: Infections and intrauterine growth retardation, Pediat. Clin North America 17:119, 1970.
13. Hytten, F. E., Paintin, D. D., Stewart, A. M., and Palmer, J. H.: The relation of maternal heart size, blood volume and stature to the birth weight of the baby, J. Obst. & Gynaec. Brit. Commonwealth 70:817, 1963.
14. James, L.: The effect of pain relief for labor and delivery on the fetus and newborn, Anesthesiology 21:405, 1960.
15. James, L. S., and Adamsons, K.: Respiratory physiology of the fetus and newborn infant, New England J. Med. 26:1352, 27:1403, 1964.

16. Lipsitz, P., and English, I.: Hyper-magnesemia in the newborn, Pediatrics 40:856, 1967.
17. Lubchenco, L. O., Hansman, C., Dressler, M., and Boyd, E.: Intrauterine growth as estimated from liveborn birthweight data at 24 to 42 weeks of gestation, Pediatrics 32:793, 1963.
18. Lubchenco, L. O.: Assessment of gestational age and development at birth, Pediat. Clin. North America 17:125, 1970.
19. Naeye, R. L., and Kelly, J. A.: Judgment of fetal age. III. The pathologist's evaluation, Pediat. Clin. North America 13:849, 1966.
20. Parmelee, A. J., Jr., Stern, E., Chervin, G., and Minkowski, A.: Gestational age and the size of premature infants, Biologia Neonatorum 6:309, 1964.
21. Pick, W.: Malnutrition of the newborn secondary to placental abnormalities, New England J. Med. 250:905, 1954.
22. Polgar, G.: The first breath: A turbulent period of physiologic adjustment, Clin. Pediat. 10:562, 1963.
23. Rossier, A., Courtois, M., and Moreux, M: Children of mothers with gravid toxemia, Ann. paediat. 37:193, 1961.
24. Scott, K. E., and Usher, R. J.: Fetal malnutrition: Its incidence, causes, and effects, Am. J. Obst. & Gynec. 94:951, 1966.
25. Smith, C. A.: The first breath, Sci. Amer. 209:27, 1963.
26. Smith, C. A.: Effect of maternal undernutrition upon the newborn infant in Holland (1944-45), J. Pediat. 30:229, 1947.
27. Usher, R. H.: Clinical and therapeutic aspects of fetal malnutrition, Pediat. Clin. North America 17:169, 1970.
28. Usher, R., McLean, F., and Scott, K. E.: Judgment of fetal age. II Clinical significance of gestational age and an objective method for its assessment, Pediat. Clin. North America 13:835, 1966.
29. Van Leeuwen, G., and Jackson, R.: Infants of diabetic mothers, Clin. Pediat. 4:315, 1965.
30. Warkany, J., Monroe, B. B., and Sutherland, B. S.: Intrauterine growth retardation, Am. J. Dis. Child. 102:249, 1961.
31. Wharton, B. A., and Bower, B. D.: Immediate or later feeding for premature babies, Lancet 2:969, 1965.

CHAPTER 3

Resuscitation of the Newborn

JOHN JONES, M.D.

Resuscitation implies re-establishing ventilation and circulation after they have ceased. Resuscitation in this text signifies the above plus the care of any newborn infant in such a way as to obviate the necessity for these extreme measures. In most newborns, adequate ventilation is the key to success. An exception might be the baby with malformation of the heart so severe as to preclude living after separation from the mother's circulation.

Oxygen is essential to animal life. Food and fluids are present in sufficient quantities so that a temporary lack causes illness but rarely death, but oxygen is not stored within the human body at any age. Even a temporary lack of oxygen can cause death. This is particularly true of the newborn, who has experienced a reduction in oxygen partial pressure during delivery. Drugs, fetal anomalies and abnormal maternal conditions add to the depression of the newborn. Any combination of these factors adds geometrically to the depression.

EVALUATION AND OBSERVATION

Proper evaluation of the infant is mandatory. The Apgar score (see Suggested Reading) is universally accepted as the standard. The usual technic is thorough evaluation within 60 seconds of birth. (Aides and L.P.N.s, as well as R.N.s and M.D.s, can evaluate the newborn, if they have been properly trained, when the obstetrician is busy with the mother.) We have found that the prognosis of a newborn is better anticipated if evaluations are made at 1 minute and again at 5 minutes of life. A rising Apgar score (e.g., a score of 4 at 1 minute and a score of 9 at 5 minutes) indicates a good prognosis, whereas a lowering of the Apgar score (e.g., a score of 8 at 1 minute and a score of 5 at 5 minutes) indicates a poor prognosis if corrective measures are not instituted. Repeti-

tive scoring at 5-minute intervals is indicated if an Apgar score of 9 or
10 has not been achieved at 10 minutes of life.

Apgar scores 0, 1 and 2—those recorded at the threshold of life—have
the following criteria:

Sign	0	1	2
Heart rate	Absent	Below 100	Above 100
Respiratory effort	Absent	Slow, irregular	Good, crying
Muscle tone	Limp	Some	Active motion
Response to nasal catheter	None	Grimace	Cough, sneeze
Color	Blue Pale	Body pink Extremities blue	Pink

Although not resuscitative measures per se, the following are observations and actions from which all newborns will benefit:

Position. Placing the baby in a slight head-down position and on its
side will help prevent intratracheal aspiration of secretions, vaginal
mucus and blood, and amniotic fluid which may be present in the
pharynx at birth.

Suctioning. During or promptly after birth the mouth, throat and
nose should be gently aspirated. Too vigorous and prolonged suctioning
should be avoided. If too vigorous, the delicate mucus membranes may
be injured, particularly in prematures. Glottic closure is a normal protective reflex when foreign materials are present above the glottis, and
the presence of the suction tip in the throat for a prolonged period will
elicit this reflex. A change in Apgar score from 8 to 5 has been observed
as a result of prolonged suctioning. An ideal program would be to suction
for 5 seconds, wait for the baby to take two or three breaths, and then
suction again, repeating this sequence until all material is removed. Obviously, if a great deal of material is present initially it will be necessary
to remove most of it before the baby can open its glottis and breathe.

Temperature. A good general rule is to keep all physiologic systems
within normal limits. This applies to newborns particularly, inasmuch

as infants are poikilothermic. The average delivery-room temperature is far below normal body temperature, so the baby loses heat rapidly unless he is placed in a warm environment. Receiving units with heating elements are a must in the delivery room. Those with a heating unit under the infant and radiant heat from above appear to be the best.

Moving the newborn. The best time to move the infant to the nursery depends upon good medical judgment and on circumstances in the hospital. The matter of least concern is keeping the infant in the delivery room for the purpose of the mother's scrutiny.

If your hospital has a newborn intensive-care nursery with trained personnel on duty around the clock and the proper equipment, the sooner you place the infant in this environment the better. If the facilities and personnel are not available, it is wise to keep the baby in the delivery room, where competent help is immediately available.

You would not consider moving an adult in shock; yet all too often we have seen neonates transferred down a long corridor as soon as possible in order to place them in isolation where an observer may not always be present. The newborn's cardiovascular system may be unstable, particularly if hypothermia, hypoxia and acidosis have been encountered, and any sudden movement will produce a decrease in cardiac output. The main problem is that the newborn is so small that it is possible to manhandle him unintentionally.

GENERAL RESPIRATORY CARE OF NEWBORN INFANTS

In general, one may consider two classes of neonates: those with an Apgar score of 5-10 and those with a score of 4 or lower.

Apgar Score of 5 to 10

1. Place the infant in a heated incubator, on his side with his head down.

2. Clear the airway with gentle intermittent suctioning.

3. Apply gentle stimulation—rubbing the back or snapping the feet may be done at this time. Vigorous stimulation—swinging, jack-knifing, compressing the chest, spanking, or dilation of the anal sphincter—should not be considered.

4. If the Apgar score is 5-7, administer oxygen by mask. Sudden flushing of oxygen over the face of the infant may elicit a cry.

5. If respiration is irregular or slow, gentle application of the mask to the face and assistance to ventilation should be instituted as soon as the airway is cleared.

6. Laryngoscopy and intubation are rarely needed in these instances unless aspiration of pharyngeal contents has already occurred.

Apgar Score of 0 to 4

1. Place the infant in a heated incubator, on his side with his head down.

2. Apply no stimulation.

3. Clear the airway with gentle, intermittent suctioning.

4. Use the infant oropharyngeal airway. Two errors in the use of the oropharyngeal airway may occur: improper insertion and wrong size. Insertion of the airway must be accomplished without pushing the tongue into the pharynx. Hold the tongue with the left index finger and slip the airway into the throat so that the tongue is held away from the posterior pharyngeal wall. Too short an airway will not accomplish this; too long an airway will impinge on the epiglottis, forcing it down over the glottic opening so as to produce a complete respiratory obstruction.

5. Apply the oxygen mask to the face and gently assist ventilation. Adequate ventilation can be ascertained by observing bilateral chest expansion and auscultating the chest, with compression of the breathing bag. Pressures of 15-20 cm. H_2O are safe for repeated inflation when properly applied; however, higher pressures may be necessary. A time-pressure relationship should be kept in mind to prevent rupturing tissues in the airway. The greater the pressure, the shorter the period of time the pressure should be applied. A bag and mask will not be suitable for inflating lungs that are completely atelectatic. The pressure necessary to inflate these lungs will exceed the opening pressure of the esophagus so that dilatation of the stomach is a complication. In this instance an endotracheal tube is preferable.

6. Laryngoscopy and intubation. When the infant has definitely aspirated material into the trachea or when the above ventilation measures are ineffective, direct larynogoscopy is indicated. A small or me-

dium handle with a straight blade is useful. Keep in mind that neonatal tissues are susceptible to trauma: gentleness is the watchword. A no. 12 French endotracheal tube may be inserted in the majority of newborns, but a no. 10 or even a no. 8 may be necessary in the very small premature. Always check by observation and auscultation to see that both lungs are being inflated.

In the event a mechanical device is not immediately at hand, puffs of air from the mouth may be used to inflate the lungs via the endotracheal tube. Only the air in the operator's mouth (not lungs) should be expelled.

7. Sodium bicarbonate (NaHCO$_3$), 1-3 mEq./kg., should be slowly administered intravenously if all the above measures have been properly taken and the baby has not responded in 3 minutes.

8. Respiratory stimulants (nikethamide, alpha-lobeline, pentylenetetrazol) are of no value, may be harmful and certainly waste time. Opiate antagonists are indicated only in case of opiate depression. Depression due to other types of drugs or other situations will be made worse by opiate antagonists.

9. Closed chest massage. In the event the heart has stopped, establish the airway and ventilation, then institute cardiac massage by compression of the midpoint of the sternum with one or two fingertips. A rate of 90/100 minutes is suitable. Repeat the sodium bicarbonate dosage (point 7, above) every 5 minutes of arrest time.

10. Suitable antibiotic therapy may be advisable after extensive resuscitation measures. Unnecessary procedures should never be done and may only delay proper therapy.

FAILURES IN RESUSCITATION

Several uncommon defects should be mentioned in relation to resuscitation, inasmuch as they may be responsible for problems in resuscitation. Although they are detailed elsewhere in this text, we will include some of them here, for completeness.

Metabolic Derangements

Hypoglycemia. Infants born of diabetic mothers may need glucose to counterbalance the excess insulin produced by the infant in utero and immediately after birth.

Hypothermia. Low body temperature slows all tissue activity, including that of the cardiovascular and respiratory systems.

Acidosis. There is significant respiratory acidosis in most newborns. When the baby has suffered prolonged hypoxia, an additional significant metabolic acidosis supervenes. Marked increase in hydrogen ion concentration is a potent depressant.

Congenital Airway Anomalies

Choanal atresia. Infants normally breathe through their nose. Choanal atresia prevents this. Application of a mask for resuscitation may approximate the lips. Should this occur in the presence of this defect, no air can pass into the lungs.

Macroglossia. An unusually large tongue can cause respiratory obstruction. Prevention of the obstruction may be obtained by placing a suture through the tongue and applying traction on the suture or by using a nasopharyngeal airway—no. 8 Portex tube cut to the proper length so that the tip lies behind the tongue in the pharynx. These temporary measures are used until definitive treatment is available.

Micrognathia. An underdeveloped mandible has the same effect as the overly large tongue and can be handled in the same fashion.

Diaphragmatic Hernia

Failure to inflate the left lung during resuscitation should lead the physician to consider this anomaly. Bowel sounds on auscultation and tympany on percussion are signs frequently found. As the infant swallows air, distention of the stomach (which may lie in the chest cavity) will give the same signs as a tension pneumothorax. A nasogastric tube prevents this complication until operative repair can be accomplished.

Spontaneous Pneumothorax

Infants have developed this problem with or without inflation of the lungs by mechanical means. Absent or diminished breath sounds plus hyper-resonance unilaterally or bilaterally with a clear airway should make one think of this possiblility. Chest tubes with an underwater seal are an immediate consideration.

Congenital Heart Disease

Most of the anomalies of the heart lead to problems after the first day of life, but some are incompatible with life.

EQUIPMENT

Suction. A De Lee or ear-bulb syringe is best. Suction from a mechanical or wall aspirator is much too traumatic for the newborn.

Airways. The Berman or Guedel premature and newborn sizes are preferred.

Endotracheal tubes. Cole tubes have been found best for the occasional user, because they have a flange 25 mm. from the tip which helps prevent insertion to too great a depth. Metric equivalents of the French sizes are as follows: no. 8, 1.5 mm.; no. 10, 2 mm.; no. 12, 2.5 mm.; no. 14, 3 mm. Cole tubes have an additional advantage: a single 4 mm. adaptor will fit all sizes.

Laryngoscope handle. A medium or small handle should be selected, because it can be grasped by the fingertips. Larger handles require grasping by the entire hand, which has the potential of a greater degree of trauma.

Laryngoscope blades. Personal preference dictates the type. A straight blade with an over-all length of 113 mm. will be satisfactory.

Self-inflating bag. There are many types. Those with a capacity of approximately 1,000 cc. and having a pop-off valve rated at 45 cm. H_2O are best.

SUGGESTED READING

Apgar, V.: A proposal for a new method of evaluation of the newborn infant, Current Res. in Anesth. & Analg. 32:260, 1953.

CHAPTER 4

Screening Procedures and Selected Malformations

G. VAN LEEUWEN, M.D.

After the infant has been transported to the nursery and after adequate ventilation and body temperature have been maintained or restored, a detailed and thorough physical examination should be performed. In addition to this examination, which is described in many other textbooks, a number of special procedures should be done in search of malformations which may not have been evident after the routine physical examination. These screening procedures have been developed primarily in three areas: hidden congenital malformations, chromosomal abnormalities and disorders of amino acid metabolism. We believe that the screening for hidden congenital anomalies should be performed on all infants, whether they are at risk or not. One should be more selective about screening for chromosomal abnormalities, and we cannot yet be very dogmatic about which infants should be screened for disorders of amino acid metabolism other than phenylketonuria. The details of the recommended procedures are given in the following pages.

CONGENITAL ANOMALY APPRAISAL

This survey, which is outlined in Table 4-1, is performed on all infants, usually within the first hour of life, and on all infants prior to the first feeding. The eyes, a stethoscope, and a soft, radiopaque no.5 or no. 8 feeding catheter are used. This series of procedures can be readily learned by a nurse. The cost of each procedure is approximately 50 cents for the catheter and syringe, and the time required is approximately 1 minute.

Table 4-1. OUTLINE OF CONGENITAL ANOMALY APPRAISAL

Procedure	Suspected Anomaly
Inquiry for polyhydraminios	Prematurity; obstructive GU and GI anomaly
Inspection of appearance of abdomen	Tumor or diaphragmatic hernia
Passage of nasogastric tube	Esophageal and choanal atresia; choanal stenosis
Aspiration of stomach, with recording of color and amount of fluid	20 ml. of yellow fluid suggests intestinal obstruction
Insertion of rectal catheter	Imperforate anus
Counting umbilical arteries	One artery suggests other anomalies, especially GU

Inquiry for Polyhydramnios

The least specific of these procedures is the inquiry about polyhydramnios. Obstetricians are often not able to provide this information accurately. The literature describes many malformations associated with polyhydramnios, and our experience confirms this: in our study approximately 40% of infants whose mothers had polyhydramnios died, and the reasons for death were extremely varied. There were obstructive genitourinary and gastrointestinal malformations, as well as extreme prematurity. Awareness of the existence of polyhydramnios alerts one to the possibility of trouble in the infant, even before delivery.

Inspection of the Abdomen

A simple inspection of the abdomen, which should be part of the routine examination, often is not. The abdomen of the normal newborn should be slightly convex. A distended abdomen suggests the presence of ascites or intra-abdominal tumor. More difficult to recognize but even more critical is the concavity of the abdominal wall, which should lead one to suspect the presence of a diaphragmatic hernia.

Passage of Nasogastric Tube

Passage of a nasogastric tube reveals a surprisingly high incidence of
choanal stenosis and unilateral choanal atresia. Our findings in 2,000 con-
secutive infants are described in Table 4-2. There is probably no significance to unilateral choanal atresia other than the knowledge of its
existence. Bilateral choanal stenosis usually gives rise to transient
respiratory distress in the neonatal period. The major significance of
this occurrence is that one need not search elsewhere for respiratory
distress. The term choanal stenosis is applied to conditions of moderate
respiratory distress not otherwise explained—provided a no. 8 catheter
cannot be passed and a no. 5 catheter can be passed only with difficulty.
Bilateral choanal atresia leads to severe respiratory distress and may require prompt surgical correction, because the newborn is an obligatory
nose-breather. We have not had to resort to tracheostomy in these infants; instead, we have been able to maintain them with an oropharyngeal airway for 2-3 days. In our hands the best airway is a standard
rubber nipple with the tip cut off. Rarely, immediate surgical correction of bilateral atresia is necessary.

When the catheter is advanced, one must be absolutely certain that
the stomach has been entered. Simple aspiration will not suffice,
because 2-3 ml. of mucus may be present in a blind esophageal pouch:

Table 4-2. CONGENITAL ANOMALIES DETECTED IN A SERIES OF 2,000 NEONATES

Major Anomalies	No. of Infants	Minor Anomalies	No. of Infants
Congenital heart disease	5	Preauricular skin tags	6
Cleft palate	2	Supernumerary digits	6
Choanal atresia or stenosis	9	Hemangioma	1
Hypospadias	4	Anal stenosis	1
Meningomyelocele	1	Umbilical hernia	9
Ambiguous genitalia	1		
Single umbilical artery (isolated)	3		
Single umbilical artery (with chromosomal trisomy)	2		
	27		23

the catheter may curl in the pouch and thus disappear but not enter the stomach. We believe the best method of being certain of having entered the stomach is to inject 1-2 ml. of air while listening with the stethoscope over the epigastrium. The noise of air entering the stomach is characteristic; and though the sound can be heard at a distance if the catheter is in the esophageal pouch, the sound will be quite distinctive. An example of a diagnosis made in the first 15 minutes of life of an esophageal atresia is shown in Figure 4-1. Because we use radiopaque catheters we do not feel it is necessary to document esophageal atresia

Fig. 4-1.—Esophageal atresia with tracheoesophageal fistula. Note the catheter outlining the esophageal pouch. The infant was 15 minutes old when this diagnosis was made.

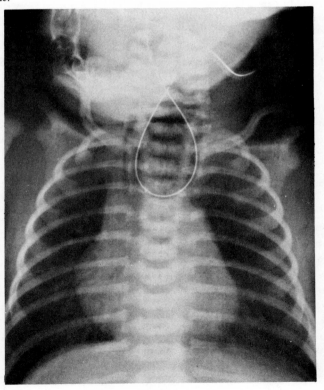

by injecting contrast material into the esophageal pouch. Not needing to do this reduces the likelihood of aspiration pneumonia.

Aspiration of the Stomach

When the stomach contents are emptied, the amount of fluid has little significance. In our series of 2,000 infants, six babies had more than 20 ml. of fluid present in the stomach but none of these had obstructive intestinal lesions. If, however, the gastric contents are bile-stained or if there is more than 30 ml. of gastric aspirate there is a need for intense observation, prompt radiologic study and informing the pediatric surgeon that the infant probably has an obstructive lesion. Infants with ileal atresia are not distended at birth, but at least the diagnosis can be highly suspected by means of the above procedure.

Insertion of Rectal Catheter

The catheter is then removed and inserted into the infant's rectum. Aspiration again takes place, and meconium should appear on the tip of the catheter. This does not absolutely indicate the presence of a patent gastrointestinal tract, but the results are nearly 100% accurate. It has been suggested that in female infants the same catheter be inserted into the vagina to determine the presence of vaginal stenosis, prior to using the catheter in the rectum. We are not certain how seriously this suggestion was meant, but we do feel that the vaginal diagnosis need not be made until sometime later in life.

Counting Umbilical Arteries

The final step in this series of procedures is a simple counting of the umbilical arteries at the point of entrance into the abdomen.

The reported incidence of single umbilical artery, as well as the frequency of a given kind of associated congenital abnormality, varies widely (Table 4-3). Some have found the incidence to be as high as 1% and associated primarily with renal anomalies: others have found the incidence to be as low as 0.2% and associated with only a small increase in anomalies over that predicted for the entire neonatal population.

Table 4-3. SUMMARY OF RECENT DATA ON SINGLE UMBILICAL ARTERY

Authors	Incidence (%)	Anomalies	
Benirschke and Brown, 1955	---	27/55	(49%)
Lenoski and Medovy, 1962	0.20	1/5	(20%)
Froehlich and Fujikura, 1966	0.76	63/203	(30.5%)
Faierman, 1960	2.70	9/11	(81.8%)
Peckham and Yerushalmy, 1965	0.90	10/51	(20%)
Benirschke and Bourne, 1960	1.00	7/15	(47%)
Lyon, 1960	1.10	2/8	(25%)
Bourne and Benirschke, 1960	---	58/113	(51%)
Little, 1961	0.75	10/21	(48%)
Cairns and McKee, 1964	1.00	2/20	(10%)
Gomori and Koller, 1964	0.80	1.8	(12.5%)
Fujikura, 1964	0.80	7/39	(18.4%)
Feingold, Fine and Ingall, 1964	0.50	15/32	(46%)
Papadatos and Paschos, 1965	0.40	10/32	(31.2%)

Many types of single and multiple anomalies have been reported in association with single umbilical artery. Most frequently recorded are those of the lower urinary tract and those in chromosomal trisomies 13-15 and 16-18. The incidence of single umbilical artery is markedly low among Negro and Oriental (Mongoloid) subjects. The incidence of single umbilical artery in twins is 3.6%, possibly as the result of disturbed placental growth; however, fetal anomalies are less common in twins than in single births with single umbilical artery.

We have studied about 7,000 infants, of whom approximately 40% were Caucasian and 60% were Negro. Most of the mothers were from the lower socioeconomic categories, but approximately 7% of them were wives of medical students and physicians. Each of the 7,000 infants received the survey for congenital anomalies within the first 60 minutes of extrauterine life, and the survey included a careful examination of the umbilical stump at the point of entry. Both arteries, when present, were identified and probed, if possible. If this could not be done by the house officer, a senior staff physician examined the stump, and a portion was sent to the laboratory for histologic examination. If only one artery was identified, a segment of the umbilical cord, from as close to skin level as possible, was fixed in 10% Formalin and submitted for histologic evaluation. Intravenous pyelograms were performed on all of these infants, as well as chromosomal karyotypes.

Table 4-4. INCIDENCE OF SINGLE UMBILICAL ARTERY AND ASSOCIATED ANOMALIES IN 4,800 CONSECUTIVELY BORN INFANTS

No. of Infants	Single Umbilical Artery	Anomalies
2,000 (Van Leeuwen and associates) (University Hospital)	6	2 Chromosomal trisomy
1,800 (Harris) (Boone County Hospital, Columbia, No.)	8	1 Hydrocephalus
1,000 (Van Leeuwen) (University Hospital)	3	0
4,800	17 (0.35%)	3

In the 17 patients of 4,800 we reported (Table 4-4), no history of the ingestion of a teratogenic drug or the occurrence of a teratogenic disease could not be elicited from any of the six mothers. Only one infant had a birth weight of less than 2,500 Gm.; his weight was 2,420 Gm. The other 16 infants were considered to be full term. All these infants were Caucasian.

Upon physical examination, 14 infants were considered to be normal, and intermittent observations of them for a period of 8-24 months revealed no abnormalities. Two infants had multiple congenital anomalies consistent with 16-18 trisomy. The existence of the trisomy was established by karyotype studies in both instances. One infant had mild arrested hydrocephalus.

We continue to recommend that the umbilical arteries be counted at birth and that intravenous pyelography be performed on infants with one artery. Beyond this, careful observation for other anomalies is advised.

PHENYLKETONURIA

A blood test for elevated concentration of phenylalanine should be performed, prior to hospital discharge, on all newborn infants after they have received milk for at least 24 hours and preferably for 48 hours.

It is recommended that a second blood test be performed on all infants at 4 to 6 weeks of age. This will detect babies who have low or borderline plasma concentrations of phenylalanine in the first few days of life, and it will serve as double insurance against false negatives.

Infants in whom there is a family history of phenylketonuria should be tested much more intensively.

The most commonly accepted laboratory test performed for phenylketonuria today is the Guthrie test. One must be careful about interpreting the results in low-birthweight infants, because they are likely to have accumulations of phenylalanine and often excrete reducing substance in the urine without having any inherited metabolic disorders. Elevated serum tyrosine is also responsible for a number of instances of positive Guthrie tests. All of these false positives must be carefully investigated so that the presence or absence of disease can be established. Screening of infants for metabolic disease is discussed in detail in Chapter 12.

MELITURIA

Every newborn should have a test for reducing substances (Clinitest) in the urine after at least 24 hours and preferably after 48 hours of milk feeding. This is a very rough screening test—it yields many false positives—but it does aid in the detection of galactosemia and hereditary fructose intolerance. It has been our policy to repeat any positives, and if a second examination is positive to go into a thorough evaluation for galactosemia and hereditary fructose intolerance. A test which measures galactose 1-phosphate uridyl transferase activity in the blood is a satisfactory screening test for galactosemia.

Many other metabolic disorders, as well as fibrocystic disease, athyrotic cretinism, etc., should be detected early; unfortunately, however, screening tests for these conditions are not yet readily applicable to all newborns. This is an important matter for investigation in the future. One hopes that ultimately the physician will have recourse to a multitude of tests to rule out all genetic and metabolic disease in the immediate neonatal period.

All infants born into a family with a history of an inherited metabolic disorder should be carefully and totally evaluated, soon after birth, by a specialist in that disorder.

CONGENITAL MALFORMATIONS

The incidence of congenital malformations is about 5% of all births. This has been confirmed by a number of studies. The majority of abnormalities are of the extremities, skin and related structures, of the spine and skull, and of the cardiovascular system. All other malformations are much less frequent. In this section we will not attempt to consider all congenital malformations but will call attention to (1) some of the more serious anomalies for which early therapy is mandatory and (2) some which may present difficulty in diagnosis.

The causes of congenital malformations are largely unknown. One can say that they fall into four categories: environmental, infectious, pharmacologic and genetic. The number of malformations for which the cause can be absolutely established, however, is probably less than 10% of the total malformations seen by the physician. Classic examples of infectious problems are, of course, congenital rubella and cytomegaloviral infections. The drugs thalidomide and 4-aminopteroyl glutamic acid (Aminopterin) are well-known teratogenic agents. The chromosomal trisomies, including mongolism, are illustrations of the genetic variety. The cause of most malformations remains unknown. We have called attention in the earlier pages of this chapter, under screening procedures, to hidden malformations. These are primarily malformations of the lungs, gastrointestinal tract and genitourinary tract. The infant may appear normal; but early diagnosis of these malformations is equally critical—in fact, in most instances is more critical. This will be emphasized throughout this section.

Malformations Requiring Immediate Attention, Sometimes Including Surgical Treatment

Head. Two of the most serious malformations requiring early intervention in the head are choanal atresia and Pierre-Robin syndrome. Newborn infants are obligatory nose-breathers, and when they have choanal atresia they will present with severe respiratory distress. A most severe example of choanal atresia is shown in Figure 4-2, in a patient who had holoprosencephaly. Choanal atresia can be diagnosed in the

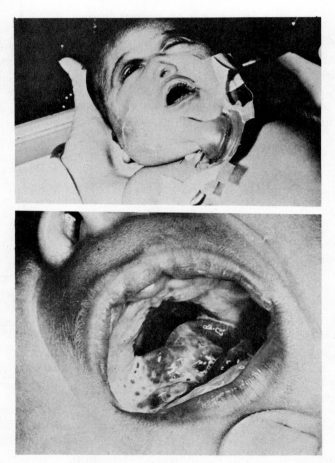

Fig. 4-2.—Baby with holoprosencephaly had a single median nasal aperture with choanal atresia. A nipple was used both as airway and for feeding.

Fig. 4-3.—Pierre-Robin syndrome: cleft palate, glossoptosis and micrognathia.

first moments of life by passage of a catheter through each side of the nose (as described in screening procedures). If choanal atresia is present, a nipple can be taped into the mouth after the end has been cut off; this can be used to help provide an airway and later to feed the infant.

If this does not suffice to keep the infant out of difficulty, surgical treatment of the choanal atresia may be mandatory in the first day or two of life.

The Pierre-Robin syndrome consists in micrognathia, cleft palate and glossoptosis (Fig.4-3)—a syndrome easily recognized. These infants may present severe respiratory distress, because the tongue falls into the opening in the palate with each attempted inspiration. Several therapeutic approaches have been advanced for this condition. We find that passing a suture as far back in the tongue as possible and crossways through it, tying the suture to the anterior lower gingival margin, is a reasonably successful method of treatment. The infant then is placed on his abdomen. The suture usually pulls out in 3-4 days, by which time the infant seems to be able to get along reasonably well. Usually, however, he has to be tube-fed for a considerable period of time. Other procedures have been described; they include tracheostomy, suturing the tongue relatively permanently to the anterior lower gingival margin, and the use of an elastic cap that suspends the infant in a position that helps the tongue fall forward. Any or all of these are acceptable.

Chest. As noted previously, cardiac malformations are relatively common in the neonate. These are discussed in detail in Chapter 5.

All infants who present with respiratory distress should, first of all, be considered to have a congenital malformation of the lungs requiring surgical attention. Although it is true that most of these infants will have either the hyaline membrane syndrome or an infectious process, the point which must be made is that they will not survive very long without surgery if they have anomalies. Examples of this kind of condition are congenital lobar emphysema (Fig. 4-4), congenital cyst of the lung (Fig. 4-5), tension pneumothorax (Fig. 4-6), diaphragmatic hernia (Fig. 4-7) and esophageal atresia with tracheoesophageal fistula (see Fig. 4-1). If the physician is faced with congenital emphysema or congenital cyst and is not able to perform definitive surgery, needles inserted into the area may be life-sustaining until surgery can be performed. Tension pneumothorax should always be treated initially with a needle; this is done with the infant sitting upright and the needle entering the apical portion of the lung at about the second interspace anteriorly. About half the time this can be treated with one needle

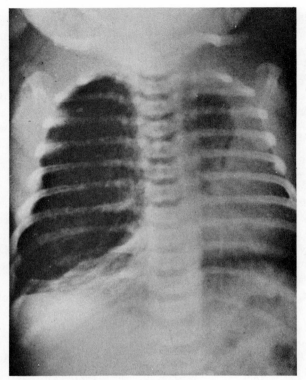

Fig. 4-4.—Example of congenital lobar emphysema of the right upper lobe. This infant weighed 4,900 Gm. and was born to a diabetic mother.

puncture. A chest x-ray should be taken 30-60 minutes after the procedure, and if the air has reaccumulated a chest tube should be inserted. The technic for chest tube insertion is described in the procedural section.

Infants with diaphragmatic hernia should have prompt surgical intervention. Their distress becomes worse as they cry and the gastrointestinal tract fills with air. For this reason inserting a tube and connecting it to low suction may significantly reduce the respiratory distress while the infant is prepared for surgical intervention.

Infants with esophageal atresia and tracheoesophageal fistula should be diagnosed before they have had any water or milk. As described under screening procedures, this can be done very simply with a nasogastric tube. If a diagnosis is made, the infant should be placed in a half-sitting position, with a catheter in the esophageal pouch on low suction. This position attempts to reduce the spilling of gastric acid contents into the bronchopulmonary tree. These infants should be operated on within 24 hours of birth; i.e., before the development of significant chemical pneumonia.

Fig. 4-5.—Demonstration of a multiloculated cyst of the lung. This patient was referred as having a diaphragmatic hernia.

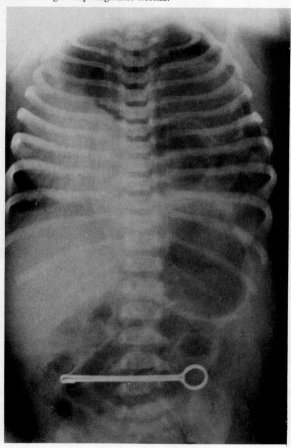

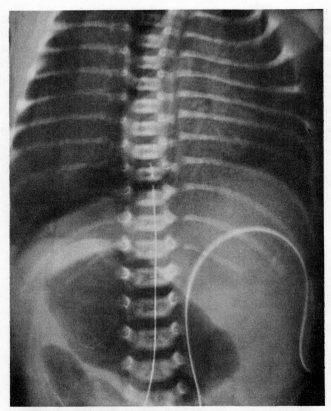

Fig. 4-6.—A 1,200 Gm. infant with tension pneumothorax on the right. The baby had been treated as having the hyaline membrane syndrome.

Gastrointestinal tract. There are several critically urgent malformations in the gastrointestinal tract besides esophageal atresia. These are meconium ileus (Fig. 4-8), ileal atresia, malrotation, volvulus and omphalocele (Fig. 4-9). Meconium ileus and ileal atresia should be suspected if more than 20 ml. of yellow fluid is present in the stomach at the time of birth. When we encounter this we promptly x-ray the infant and alert our surgical colleagues, whose help may be needed. Meconium ileus is almost always associated with cystic fibrosis of the pancreas. If diagnosed very early, meconium ileus is sometimes successfully relieved by a Mucomyst enema or a trypsin-containing enema, in an attempt to produce passage of the meconium; but if the infant is more than a few hours old, these procedures simply waste valuable time, and an operation should be done. Our own experience with meconium ileus has been very discouraging: those infants who have survived the ileus have almost always succumbed to cystic fibrosis at 3 or 4 years of age. Ileal atresia, on the other hand, carries with it an excellent prognosis— if the diagnosis is made before the infant is fed milk and has the opportunity to vomit, aspirate and become dehydrated. The survival is directly related to the early diagnosis and to the skill of the surgeon.

Fig. 4-7.—Massive diaphragmatic hernia on the left. The stomach and most of the small intestine were in the chest cavity.

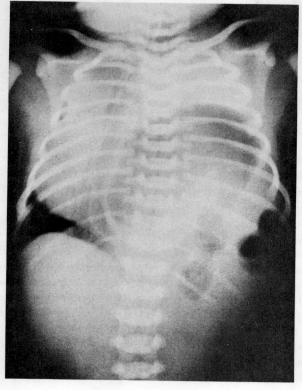

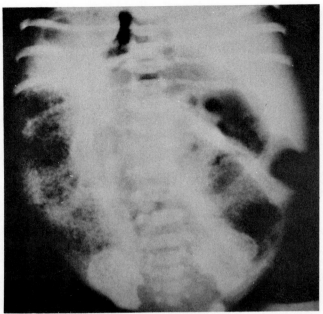

Fig. 4-8.—Meconium ileus in a first-born infant. There was no family history of cystic fibrosis of the pancreas. Note the markedly distended loops of bowel.

Malrotation may be present alone and asymptomatic for life, or it may become symptomatic because volvulus supervenes. Volvulus may occur in an apparently normal bowel or in a malrotated bowel. It is frequently a complication of meconium ileus and of duplication of the bowel. Good prognosis and survival depend on early diagnosis and immediate operative correction. Diagnosis rests on sudden onset of vomiting and rapid development of distention. Cases have been reported as early as the third or fourth day and as late as a month or more. Operative treatment is imperative not so much because of high intestinal obstruction as because of the rapid development of gangrene.

An omphalocele is easily recognized. The sac should be kept moist and as sterile as possible until surgical intervention can be performed. There are many surgical approaches to this lesion, including the treatment of the entire area with silver nitrate in an attempt to promote granulation, to complete reduction and repair.

Central nervous system. The two conditions which require most prompt treatment in the central nervous system are meningomyelocele (Fig. 4-10) and sacrococcygeal teratoma (Figs. 4-11 and 4-12). In recent years, since the meningomyelocele has been covered with skin in the first 12 to 24 hours of life, the survival rate as well as the mental function of these infants has greatly improved. Meningomyeloceles should be covered and kept sterile until a neurosurgeon can be consulted. We believe these should be considered surgical emergencies and immediately repaired.

Hydrocephalus usually follows. This is treated with shunting (discussed later).

Sacrococcygeal teratoma is almost always benign at birth but has a very high incidence of malignant degeneration if left untreated. Most of these tumors are large, and they are removed surgically just because of the size of the mass. In some instances the mass is small and therefore is overlooked; it may undergo malignant degeneration, particularly after six months of age.

Extremities. Clubfoot requires relatively prompt attention. Casting is important from very early onset to insure that the foot ultimately will be normal.

Congenital dislocation of the hip is difficult to diagnose in the neonatal period, particularly if it is bilateral. A number of signs have been described; they include telescoping (Orlando's sign). Most of the

Fig. 4-9.—Omphalocele containing liver, stomach and duodenum. This was gradually closed with mesh, with a good result.

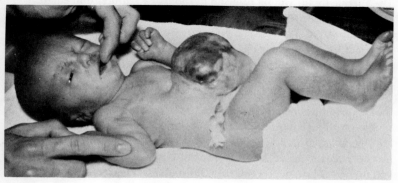

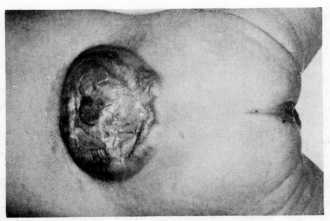

Fig. 4-10.—Newborn with a large lumbar meningomyelocele.

signs demonstrate the inability to abduct the hip to 90 degrees. We believe that most hips are only subluxated in the neonatal period, and this is why they are so frequently overlooked. The diagnosis should always be made, however, by 6 weeks of age: treatment instituted at that date usually will result in a normal hip.

Skin. The most serious abnormality of the skin requiring prompt attention is actually a hematologic disorder. It is best illustrated by Fig. 4-13, showing a twin-to-twin transfusion. There may be extreme anemia secondary to bleeding into the mother; or else the infant may be extremely polycythemic. Either condition requires immediate therapy. The anemic infant will be pale and in shock, he requires immediate blood transfusion, because in many instances the shock becomes irreversible within 2 hours. The polycythemic infant, on the other hand, is subject to cerebral thrombosis, hyperbilirubinemia and hypoglycemia, and therefore if symptomatic should be treated with a modified exchange transfusion with low-hematocrit blood. In our nursery hematocrits are done on all infants in the first hour of life, so that neither of these possibilities may be overlooked.

Eye. Although rare, both congenital glaucoma and retinoblastoma are emergency situations in the neonatal period. Congenital glaucoma can best be recognized by the observation of a cloudy, steaming cornea and increased intraocular pressure. Retinoblastoma can be detected only

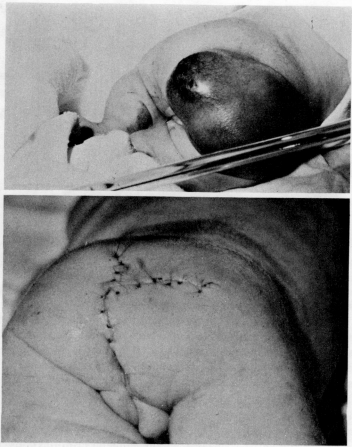

Fig. 4-11.—Sacrococcygeal teratoma. This tumor was removed at 2 days of age (see Fig. 4-12). All tumors of this type should be removed early.
Fig. 4-12.—Same patient as in Figure 4-11, after operation.

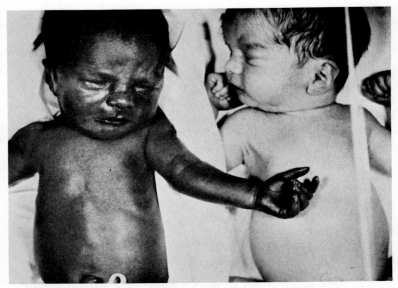

Fig. 4-13.—Twin-to-twin transfusion. The baby on the left presented with a hematocrit of 85%; the one on the right was in shock, with a hematocrit of 20%.

if a careful funduscopic examination is done on each infant. We find it easier to do this on the third day of life, when the infant is being discharged and the edema secondary to silver nitrate instillation has diminished.

Other Important Malformations

Cleft lip and palate is one of the more common malformations. The infant appears grotesque, but treatment is very satisfactory. We have concerned ourselves primarily with the lip, which we believe should be repaired at the earliest possible time. When the infant is gaining weight and has been carefully examined for other malformations, the lip should be repaired. We do not teach these infants to suck; instead, they receive cup feedings from the beginning, so that scar-enlarging tension will not be placed on the surgical repair site. Repairing of the palate is left up to the surgeon but is now done at a much earlier age than previously.

Macroglossia. A typical example of macroglossia is seen in the infant with Beckwith's syndrome (Fig. 4-14). These infants also have abnormalities of the umbilicus, hypoglycemia and large livers, and they frequently have Wilm's tumor. Macroglossia should always make one suspect mongolism, hypothyroidism, and Beckwith's syndrome.

Cystic hygroma occurs most often in the cervical region (Fig. 4-15) but also may occur in the axilla. This should be corrected promptly. The operation is often difficult, because the tumor involves and surrounds the facial nerve. The particular one illustrated in Figure 4-15 also extended down into the lung but was well encapsulated there. Cystic hygroma has a marked tendency to recur.

Fig. 4-14.—Hyperplastic visceromegaly (Beckwith's syndrome), demonstrating macroglossia.

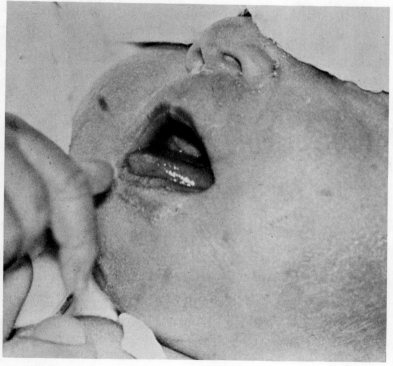

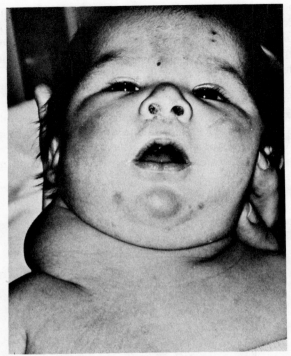

Fig. 4-15.—Cystic hygroma in the neck region. This mass extended into the thoracic cavity.

Bladder exstrophy is usually associated with severe epispadias and has a very dismal prognosis. Genitourinary surgeons should be promptly contacted, but the results are very unsatisfactory. Operation is possible; it is intended to close the abdominal wall and transplant the urethral orifice into the ileum.

Adrenogenital syndrome. Recognizing the adrenogenital syndrome is important for two reasons: (1) so that the child may be properly identified sexually, and (2) to recognize the possiblity of salt-losing syndrome. Hypertrophy of the clitoris in female infants may be so extensive that the child is incorrectly interpreted as a male (Fig. 4-16). Diagnosis depends on chromosomal sex determinations from buccal mucosa smears, best done after 3 weeks of age. Measurement of 17-

ketosteroid excretion is helpful, although it may not be elevated in the first few days. Occasionally the infant is insulted with a low sodium chloride intake to attempt to induce the salt-losing episode prior to dismissal from the hospital. In the salt-losing situations, the babies can become terminal so rapidly that this insult is felt to be justified.

Phocomelia (Fig. 4-17) has been associated primarily with the ingestion of the drug thalidomide. In other instances the cause usually is undetermined. Babies with phocomelia can be fitted with prosthetic devices very early in life. One should attempt to avoid all drugs during pregnancy, because it is unknown which drugs may produce deformities. Other abnormalities of the limbs which are very common include polydactylism and syndactylism.

Achondroplasia. The achondroplasic dwarf can readily be recognized in the neonatal period because of the relatively large head, normal trunk and very short extremities. It should be understood that hydrocephalus is common in achondroplastic dwarfs but that the children are usually mentally normal and the hydrocephalus is self-arresting.

Fig. 4-16.—Female infant with salt-losing type of virilizing adrenal hyperplasia. The family physician incorrectly called the baby a male with hypospadias.

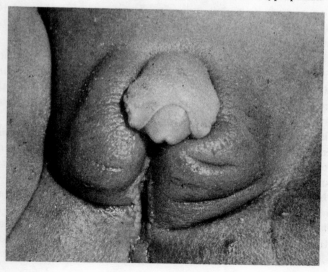

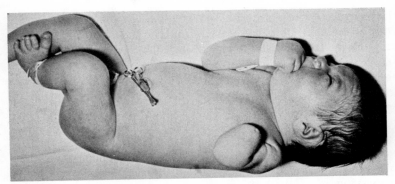

Fig. 4-17.—Infant of a diabetic mother with a large portion of the left upper extremity absent. In addition to insulin and vitamins prescribed by her physician, this mother ingested multiple drugs for her "nerves," "appetite," etc.

Hydrocephalus is of primary concern to us from a prevention standpoint. The infant who has had a meningomyelocele repaired usually develops hydrocephalus, and this can be controlled or prevented by the insertion of a ventriculoatrial shunt. Hydrocephalus which has been acquired in utero has a very poor prognosis and often results in early death.

Arthrogryposis multiplex congenita. This rare disorder (Fig. 4-18) consists of flexion deformities of one or more joints, with hypoplasia of related muscles. Treatment consists primarily in physiotherapy. Prognosis is reasonably good for general development, although the improvement of the extremities is limited. The baby shown in Figure 4-18 also had osteogenesis imperfecta, which resulted in multiple fractures at birth. This infant expired in the first few days of life from respiratory distress syndrome.

Malformations of the skin are common and do not usually require any kind of treatment. Vascular nevi appear in one form or another on almost all infants. Only if a vascular nevus is large enough to produce an associated thrombocytopenia is therapy necessary. Occasionally, if the orbit is involved, therapy is also necessary. Many of these nevi are absent at birth but appear in the first few weeks of life.

Aplasia cutis congenita (Fig. 4-19), or cutaneous defect of the scalp, is relatively common. Usually it is located near the midline of the skull. These lesions should not be treated; instead, they should be allowed to granulate. Surgical closure has been reported to result in a high incidence of brain abscess.

Congenital ichthyosis, or collodion skin, is an uncommon condition usually incompatible with life: these infants usually die in 2-3 days. The condition is familial and is most common in the males. A severe form of congenital ichthyosis is shown in Figure 4-20.

A host of other skin abnormalities—preauricular tags and sinuses, branchial cysts, etc.—are readily recognized, are not serious and require minimal therapy.

Chromosomal malformations. Down's syndrome (mongolism) is a well-described entity consisting primarily of mongoloid slant to the eyes, fullness of the neck, hypermobility of the joints, short fifth finger and single transverse palmar crease (Fig. 4-21). It is often associated with congenital heart disease. This syndrome is either a trisomy of the 17-21 group or a translocation in this group. Infants who have the translocation variety have parents who are carriers; infants with trisomy have normal

Fig. 4-18.—Three-day-old baby with arthrogryposis multiplex congenita and probable osteogenesis imperfecta. There were flexion deformities of the elbows, wrists, fingers, hips and toes. Fractures were present in both humeri and in the right femur.

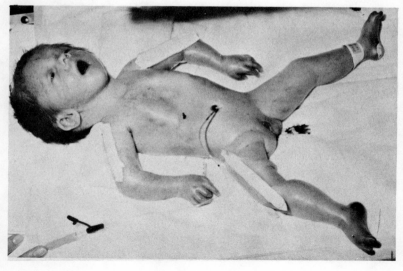

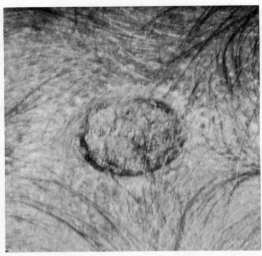

Fig. 4-19.—Aplasia cutis congenita of the scalp. These lesions are usually near the midline. This lesion had partially healed by granulation before birth.

Fig. 4-20.—Severe congenital ichthyosis is responsible for the so-called harlequin fetus. This baby died at 3 days of age.

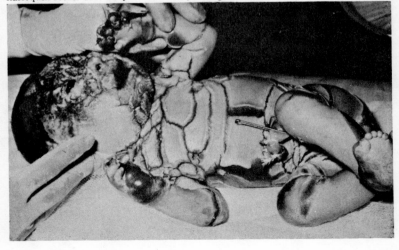

chromosome-karyotype parents. The diagnosis should always be made in the first few days of life but it is frequently overlooked. The diagnosis may be difficult in the first day or two, when the infant's eyes are edematous, but thereafter is rather easily made.

All of the chromosomal trisomies have in common the fact that mental retardation accompanies chromosomal aberration. For this reason treatment is unsatisfactory. The heart disease present in mongolism is often severe and may result in early death. Some children with this dis-

Fig. 4-21.—Classic facial appearance in Down's syndrome (mongolism). Note the slanting of the eyes.

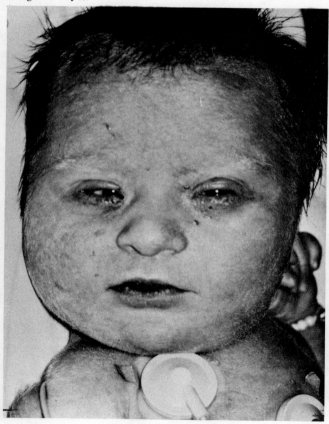

order, however, grow up to lead relatively useful lives, if they are properly stimulated and not institutionalized.

Trisomy 13-15 (Fig. 4-22) and trisomy 16-18 (Fig. 4-23) have in common mental retardation, abnormalities of the jaw and palate, abnormalities of the hands and feet, ambiguous genitalia and congenital heart disease. The most characteristic difference between the two is that in 13-15 trisomy—a very rare condition—the eyes are abnormal. This is illustrated in Figure 4-22. On the other hand, 16-18 trisomy is likely to have more severe congenital heart disease, and the infant usually expires in the first few months of life. There is one recorded incidence of a child 4 years old with 16-18 trisomy. Recently a significant increase in patients with 16-18 trisomy has been noted.

Fig. 4-22.—A 13-15 trisomy showing unilateral anophthalmia, micrognathia, abnormal right ear, and cyst on forehead.

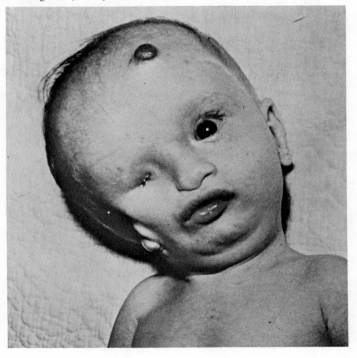

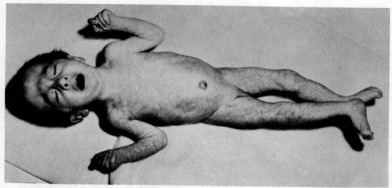

Fig. 4-23.—A 16-18 trisomy showing classic flexion of hands, cyanosis related to the congenital heart lesion, and micrognathia.

Many new entities show partial deletions of the 16-18 chromosome group. This is associated with all types of malformations. Chromosomal karyotyping is mandatory for any infant who has congenital anomalies that are not clearly understood, or who has a very unusual appearance. There are, undoubtedly, many types of chromosomal abnormalities which have not yet been detected.

The cat cry syndrome is associated with a partial deletion of the long arm of the fourth or fifth chromosome pair. The infant characteristically is long and thin. Because of associated laryngeal weakness his cry is very similar to the mewing of a cat. The long-term prognosis is reasonably good, but there is mental retardation.

Other anomalies. Every congenital malformation, no matter how minor, carries with it the obvious implication that the embryo was insulted. It logically follows that all infants with one anomaly should be suspected of, and in most instances investigated for, other malformations.

SUGGESTED READINGS

1. Apgar, V., James, L. S., and Smith, M.: *Diagnosis of Hidden Congenital Anomalies* (New York: National Foundation—March of Dimes, 1960).
2. Benirschke, K., and Bourne, G. L.: The incidence and prognostic implication of congenital absence of one umbilical artery, Am. J. Obst. & Gynec. 79:251, 1960.

3. Benirschke, K., and Brown, W. H.: Vascular anomaly of umbilical cord, Obst. & Gynec. 6:399, 1955.
4. Benirschke, K.: Editorial Comment, in Gellis, S. S. (ed.): *Year Book of Pediatrics,* 1963-64 Series (Chicago: Year Book Medical Publishers, 1964), p. 5.
5. Benirschke, K.: Major Pathologic Features of the Placenta, Cord and Membranes, in *Symposium on the Placenta* (New York: National Foundation, 1965), p. 52.
6. Bourne, G. L., and Benirschke, K.: Absent umbilical artery, a review of 113 cases, Arch. Dis. Childhood 35:534, 1960.
7. Cairns, J. D., and McKee, J.: Single umbilical artery, Canad. M.A.J. 91:1017, 1964.
8. Faierman, E.: The significance of one umbilical artery, Arch. Dis. Childhood 35:285, 1960.
9. Feingold, M., Fine, R. N., and Ingall, D.: Intravenous pyelography in infants with single umbilical artery. A preliminary report, New England J. Med. 270:1178, 1964.
10. Froehlich, L. A., and Fujikura, T.: Significance of a single umbilical artery, Am. J. Obst. & Gynec. 94:274, 1966.
11. Fujikura, T.: Single umbilical artery and congenital malformations, Am. J. Obst. & Gynec. 86:829, 1964.
12. German, J. L., Rankin, J. K., Harrison, P. A., Donovan, D. J., Hogan, W. J., and Bearn, A. G.: Autosomal trisomy of a group 16-18 chromosome, J. Pediat. 60:503, 1962.
13. Gomori, V. Z., and Koller, T.: Über das Fehlen einer Arterie in der Nabelschnur, Gynaecologia 157:177, 1964.
14. Green, C. R.: The frequency of maldevelopment in man, Am. J. Obst. & Gynec. 90:994, 1964.
15. Harris, L., and Steinburg, A.: Abnormalities observed during the first six days of life in 8,716 live-born infants, Pediatrics 14:314, 1954.
16. Lenoski, E. F., and Dedovy, H.: Single umbilical artery. Incidence, clinical significance and relation of autosomal trisomy, Canad. M.A.J. 87:1229, 1962.
17. Lewis, D. J.: Autosomal trisomy, Lancet 1:866, 1962.
18. Little, W. A.: Umbilical artery aplasia, Obst. & Gynec. 17:695, 1961.
19. Lyon, F. A.: Fetal abnormalities associated with umbilical cords containing one umbilical artery and one umbilical vein, Obst. & Gynec. 16:719, 1960.
20. McIntosh, R., Merritt, K., Richards, M. R., Samuels, M. H., and Bellows, M. T.: The incidence of congenital malformations: A study of 5,964 pregnancies, Pediatrics 14:505, 1954.

21. Mellin, G.: The Fetal Life Study of the Columbia Presbyterian Medical Center, in Chipman, S., Lilienfeld, A., Greenberg, B., and Donnelly, J. (ed.): *Research Methodology and Needs in Perinatal Studies* (Springfield, Ill.: Charles C Thomas, Publisher, 1966), p. 88.
22. Miller, J. Q., Picard, E. H., Alkau, M. K., Warner, S., and Gerald, P. S.: A specific congenital brain defect in 13-15 trisomy, New England J. Med. 268:120, 1963.
23. Moya, F., Apgar, V., James, S., and Berrien, C.: Hydramnios and congenital anomalies, J.A.M.A. 171:1552, 1960.
24. Papadatos, C., and Paschos, A.: Single umbilical artery and congenital malformations, Obst. & Gynec. 26:367, 1965.
25. Peckham, C. H., and Yerushalmy, J.: Aplasia of one umbilical artery: Incidence by race and certain obstetric factors, Obst. & Gynec. 26:359, 1965.
26. Priman, J.: Anastomosis of the umbilical arteries, Anat. Rec. 134:1, 1959.
27. Scriver, C. R.: Methods available for largescale screening programmes, Pediat. Clin. North America 12:812, 1965.
28. Seki, M., and Strauss, L.: Absence of one umbilical artery, Arch. Path. 78:446, 1964.
29. Uchida, I. A., Bowman, J. M., and Wang, H. C.: The 18-trisomy syndrome, New England J. Med. 266:1198, 1962.
30. Van Leeuwen, G., Behringer, B., and Glenn, L.: Single umbilical artery, J. Pediat. 71:103, 1967.
31. Van Leeuwen, G., and Glenn, L.: Screening for hidden congenital anomalies, Pediatrics 71:147, 1968.

CHAPTER 5

Respiratory Problems

ELIZABETH JAMES, M.D.

Respiratory problems of the newborn can be immediately life-threatening; therefore they demand prompt diagnostic and therapeutic efforts on the part of the physician. Diagnosis must be emphasized, because treatment of respiratory difficulty varies markedly with the etiology of that difficulty. For this reason we will approach the broad subject of respiratory problems of the newborn from a patient-oriented point of view, first stressing diagnostic clues and then considering methods of treatment.

UPPER AIRWAY OBSTRUCTION

The infant who presents with high obstructive symptoms is generally easily identified. Vigorous but ineffective inspiratory efforts may be made, as is usually the case with laryngeal atresia; or the infant is apneic from birth. Auscultation of the chest quickly identifies ineffective respiratory efforts.

The infant with choanal atresia may ventilate well while crying (mouth open) but be in severe difficulty otherwise, because the newborn is a nose-breather. Relief of symptoms resulting from manual opening of the mouth and inability to pass a nasal catheter (no. 5 French feeding tube) virtually make the diagnosis. If it is impossible to pass a no. 8 French nasal catheter and a no. 5 passes only with difficulty, choanal stenosis should be suspected and the infant must be observed closely for later signs of obstruction. If one is in doubt about the patency of one of the posterior choanae, observation of the child while first one and then the other external naris is held shut will reveal whether it is possible for air to pass. In the event that an oral airway is necessary, a temporary one may be easily devised by cutting off the tip of a rubber nipple and placing the nipple in the infant's mouth, taking care to secure it by attaching heavy string to two opposite sides of the base of the nipple and tying the string behind the baby's head.

Reserpine given to the mother as long as 2 days before delivery can produce the so-called stuffy nose syndrome in the infant. Such a child presents with nasal discharge, retractions and cyanosis. An oral airway is the treatment of choice, because the problem disappears in 1-5 days.

Cysts and tumors in the nose, mouth, pharynx or neck are less common causes of upper airway obstruction. Aberrant thyroid may present in this manner, as may macroglossia and congenital goiter.

The Pierre-Robin syndrome, a combination of micrognathia, glossoptosis and cleft palate, may present with obstructive signs, which are relieved by pulling the tongue forward, by using an oral airway or by placing the child on his abdomen so that the tongue falls forward and no longer obstructs the airway. Variants of the syndrome with intact palate present in the same manner. Rarely, surgical fusion of the tongue to the lower lip may be necessary.

Congenital stridors, recognized by their characteristic crowing inspiration, have numerous causes: laryngeal webs and cysts, subglottic stenosis, tracheal stenosis, vascular rings which result in tracheal compression, vocal cord paralysis and simple laryngeal stridor ("laryngomalacia"). Differentiation of these various causes is made by direct laryngoscopy or by radiographic contrast studies.

HYALINE MEMBRANE DISEASE AND OTHER DISORDERS WITH SIMILAR CLINICAL PICTURES

The remaining and most frequent causes of respiratory difficulty tend to present with a similar clinical picture: dyspnea, tachypnea, retractions, grunting and varying degrees of inadequate oxygenation as manifested by cyanosis.

It should be pointed out that cyanosis does not necessarily indicate pulmonary disease. Congenital heart disease or hypothermia may present with cyanosis, with or without tachypnea; cyanosis without dyspnea suggests intracranial problems. Gastric perforation may present with cyanosis and respiratory embarrassment.

To assume that every baby with grunting, tachypnea and retractions has hyaline membrane disease can be a fatal mistake, because many causes of such a picture are surgically or metabolically correctable. Hypoglycemia may present with tachypnea, as can severe blood loss or polycythemia. It therefore follows that any infant with respiratory difficulty of this sort should have his blood glucose concentration and hematocrit determined at once.

In order to differentiate anatomic and infectious causes of respiratory distress from hyaline membrane disease, the early obtaining of a chest x-ray (posterior-anterior and lateral) is mandatory. Conditions which can generally be diagnosed or at least suspected by obtaining chest x-rays include the following: diaphragmatic hernia, diaphragmatic eventration, diaphragmatic paralysis, pneumothorax, pneumomediastinum, lobar emphysema, and cysts and tumors. Aspiration syndromes, pulmonary hemorrhage, pneumonia and hyaline membrane disease may at times exhibit similar x-ray abnormalities. History and other factors usually help to differentiate these, however.

The importance of obtaining a good history cannot be overemphasized. Prolonged rupture of membranes, prolonged labor and fever in the mother suggest bacterial pneumonia, and the presence of maternal polyhydramnios suggests tracheoesophageal fistula with esophageal atresia, other gastrointestinal obstructive problems or maternal diabetes.

Table 5-1 lists the causes of respiratory distress which may clinically resemble hyaline membrane disease.

Hyaline Membrane Disease

Clinical picture. The infant with hyaline membrane disease is typically prematurely born, appropriate for his gestational age or, in the case of an infant of a diabetic mother, large for his gestational age. There is often, but not invariably, a history of perinatal asphyxia. Close observation shows that most affected infants have some respiratory difficulty immediately after birth. The remainder develop tachypnea, retractions and expiratory grunting within the first few hours of life. The expiratory grunt, perhaps described more appropriately as a complaining cry or whimper, is associated with increased intrathoracic pressure and is

Table 5-1. CAUSES OF RESPIRATORY DISTRESS WHICH MAY RESEMBLE HYALINE MEMBRANE DISEASE

Congenital anomalies
    Tracheoesophageal fistula
    Diaphragmatic hernia
    Diaphragmatic eventration
    Pulmonary agenesis and hypoplasia
    Lobar emphysema
    Pulmonary cysts
    Cystic adenomatoid malformation of the lung
    Other intrathoracic cysts and tumors
    Pulmonary lymphangiectasis

Infections
    Bacterial and viral pneumonias

Aspiration syndromes
    Meconium, amniotic fluid, vaginal contents

Pulmonary hemorrhage

Pneumothorax

Pneumomediastinum

Diaphragmatic paralysis

Chylothorax and pleural effusion

Transient tachypnea of the newborn

a protective type of breathing which increases the arterial oxygen tension. The mechanism by which this is accomplished is uncertain but may involve improvement in alveolar ventilation.

As the disease progresses, dyspnea increases and cyanosis appears. The lower sternum is depressed, and the upper chest is prominent. Breath sounds are generally harsh and may diminish in intensity as the disease continues. Percussion of the premature's chest is, in general, unrewarding because of the wide transmission of sounds over the small volume involved.

Poor prognostic signs include apneic episodes alternating with periods of very rapid breathing, a fixed heart rate (110-120/minute) and progressive cyanosis.

Chest x-rays show a diffuse finely reticulogranular opacification throughout both lung fields with a superimposed air bronchogram.

In fatal cases, death usually occurs before 3 days of age. Those who will recover have clearly shown improvement by 3-5 days.

Pathogenesis. The pathogenesis of hyaline membrane disease has been the subject of much speculation since the disease was first described. For a review of the existing theories, the reader is referred to Nelson's consideration of the etiology of hyaline membrane disease (see Suggested Readings). The existence of numerous theories in itself suggests that many factors are operative. Figure 5-1 illustrates the complexity of factors which influence the development and course of the disease.

Principles of treatment. From a knowledge of those factors which influence the disease we see that certain therapeutic and preventive measures are appropriate:

1. Maternal hypoxia, hypotension and decreased uterine blood flow should be avoided before delivery.

2. Prompt resuscitation is indicated in those infants in need of respiratory assistance in the delivery room.

3. Hypothermia in the infant should be constantly guarded against, because chilling is known to increase pulmonary vasoconstriction and acidosis.

4. The premature infant should not be denied his normal placental transfusion. Cord clamping can usually be delayed until the infant has taken several breaths.

Fig. 5-1.—Interrelationships of factors influencing hyaline membrane disease. (Adapted from Chu, J., et al.: Preliminary report: The pulmonary hypoperfusion syndrome, Pediatrics 35:733, 1965.)

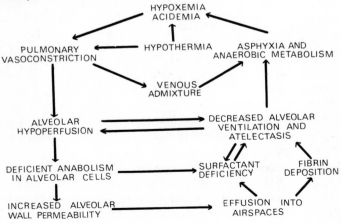

5. Adequate oxygenation and prompt correction of acidosis with sodium bicarbonate infusions promotes pulmonary vasodilatation in affected infants. Ventilation should be facilitated by placing the infant on his back, with his shoulders slightly elevated.

6. Shock should be treated immediately with blood transfusions. It should also be remembered that a packed cell volume of 40% represents significant anemia in the newborn.

7. Antibiotics should be given if there is a likelihood that infection is present.

These are general principles. Several aspects of treatment are considered in more detail in the following sections.

Monitoring. Constant monitoring of the infant with respiratory distress is essential. Heart rate, respiratory rate and the incidence of apneic episodes must be known so that intelligent decisions can be made as to therapy. It is useful to plot these variables, along with P_{O_2}, P_{CO_2} and pH values, on a bedside graph so that the effects of environmental temperature, bicarbonate infusions, change in inspired oxygen concentration, etc., may be more easily seen. Measurement of blood pressure by a pressure transducer attached to the umbilical artery catheter is also extremely helpful. Arterial pressures of less than 35-40 mm. Hg should be treated with transfusions of fresh whole blood.

Thermoregulation. It has already been pointed out that chilling increases pulmonary vasoconstriction and promotes acidosis; therefore it can be expected to adversely affect the infant with hyaline membrane disease. However, it is also important not to minimize metabolic expenditures in the sick infants. It should not be erroneously assumed that the environmental temperature is proper as long as the baby's body temperature remains normal. Most babies can maintain a normal temperature even when subjected to marked cold stress; however, the infant maintains that temperature at great metabolic expense. It is only when his defenses have been overwhelmed that the rectal temperature falls.

The thermoneutral zone is defined as that range of temperature at which the infant's metabolism is minimal. Raising or lowering the temperature outside this zone results in a rise in metabolic rate. The infant already having respiratory distress is then forced to further increase his oxygen consumption, and the demand may precipitate respiratory failure.

For a 2-kg. infant in the first day of life the thermoneutral zone is
34-34.5°C.; for a 1-kg. infant, 35-35.5°C. Humidity should be maintained at 50%. Hey and Katz (see Suggested Readings) have devised a
useful graph showing the range of temperatures necessary to provide
neutral environmental conditions during the newborn period.

Oxygen therapy. The baby receiving oxygen therapy must have that
therapy carefully monitored, and the inspired oxygen concentration
must be recorded. The arterial P_{O_2} must be checked every 4-6 hours
while supplemental oxygen is being administered to the infant whose
clinical condition is changing. It is essential to keep a bedside record of
the amount of blood withdrawn for various studies, so that appropriate
replacement may be made.

Arterialized capillary blood is not reliable for the determination of
arterial P_{O_2}: it has been shown that such measurements do not agree
with simultaneous measurements on arterial blood. Arterial samples are
most easily obtained from an indwelling catheter placed in the umbilical artery. Alternatively, arterial blood may be obtained from a radial
or temporal artery puncture. It should be remembered that blood obtained from the abdominal aorta is postductal blood and may have a
lower oxygen tension than the blood supplying the retinas, if a right-
to-left shunt is present. The inspired oxygen concentration should be
adjusted to keep the P_{O_2} as measured via the umbilical artery catheter
between 60 and 80 mm. Hg. It is particularly important to repeat
measurements after administration of alkalis, which may lower pulmonary vascular resistance and decrease right-to-left shunts, and to take frequent measurements during the recovery phase of respiratory distress,
when arterial oxygen tensions may suddenly rise as shunts diminish
and subject the infant to the risk of retrolental fibroplasia.

It may be possible to raise the arterial P_{O_2} in those infants showing
progressive worsening of blood gases by providing a positive-pressure
environment. Oxygen is allowed to flow into a plastic bag surrounding
the infant's head; the bag's outlet is attached to an underwater seal so
that oxygen pressure greater than 7-10 cm. H_2O is bubbled off. This may
be more effective when the positive pressure is supplied via a T tube
attached to an endotracheal tube. The need for respirator therapy may
thereby be avoided.

Fluid therapy. Fluid therapy in the infant with respiratory distress
has several purposes: maintenance of hydration, providing of calories,

prevention of hypoglycemia and correction of acidosis. All of these are achieved by infusion of a 10% dextrose solution with added alkali at a rate of 65-70 ml./kg. per day during the first days of life.

It is advisable to use, initially, one fourth to one half of the amount calculated to correct the total base deficit and re-evaluate the acidosis before additional base is given. (Base excess may be calculated once the pH and P_{CO_2} have been determined.) When base excess (negative base excess = base deficit) is used for calculation of the amount of base required for correction, the following equation may be used:

$$\text{mEq. base required} = \text{negative base excess}\,(\text{mEq./L.}) \times \text{weight (kg.)} \times 0.3$$

Half the amount calculated in this manner will give approximately one-fourth correction, and it should be given over a period of 20-30 minutes as a dilute solution. (It must be remembered that the commercially available sodium bicarbonate solution, containing 44.6 mEq./50 ml., is a hypertonic solution and must be given slowly in at least a 1:1 dilution.) The remaining deficit can then be replaced over a period of 3-6 hours. As a rule of thumb, the total bicarbonate given should not exceed 12 mEq./kg. per day. Serum sodium levels must be monitored at least daily while therapy is being given.

Persistent severe acidosis may require treatment with tris(hydroxymethyl)aminomethane (THAM) to avoid hypernatremia. When 0.3-M THAM is used, the above equation reduces to:

$$\text{ml. THAM required} = \text{weight (kg.)} \times \text{negative base excess}$$

One fourth of this dose is given in 5% dextrose over 20-30 minutes, and a second fourth is given over 3-6 hours. The pH, P_{CO_2} and base excess must be monitored hourly, and the amount of THAM given must be adjusted accordingly. Side effects of THAM include apnea, hypoglycemia and vascular irritation. It must only be given when the patient is being mechanically ventilated or when apparatus for mechanical ventilation is immediately available; it must be given via a large vessel (other than the umbilical vein, because liver necrosis can result from infusion into the liver); and blood glucose levels must be monitored closely.

If it is not possible to determine P_{CO_2} and base excess figures are therefore not available, sodium bicarbonate may be added to the parenteral fluids in proportion to the degree of acidosis as estimated by arterial blood pH. If the pH is between 7.2 and 7.3, 5 mEq. sodium bicarbonate per 100 ml. of 10% dextrose is given at 65-70 ml./kg. per day; 10 mEq./100 ml. is given if the pH is between 7.1 and 7.2; and 15 mEq./ 100 ml. is given if the pH is below 7.1.

For a more detailed consideration of acid-base measurements and alkali therapy, the articles by Behrman and Strauss, listed in the Selected Readings, are recommended.

Respirators. Assisted ventilation should be undertaken only by an experienced and organized intensive-care team. The type of respirator used depends mostly on the experience of the team. Indications for initiation of mechanical ventilation include an aortic P_{O_2} of less than 30-40 mm. Hg when the infant is breathing 100% oxygen, persistent elevation of arterial P_{CO_2} above 70 mm. Hg or prolonged apnea unresponsive to any stimulation.

Sudden respiratory failure may result from intracranial hemorrhage or from a pneumothorax. Immediate chest x-ray should always be obtained in such a case.

Meconium Aspiration

At the time of delivery of a meconium-stained infant with signs of upper airway obstruction, the larynx should be visualized immediately with a laryngoscope and any obstructing meconium should be suctioned. Positive-pressure resuscitation should not precede removal of meconium.

The clinical picture of the infant who has aspirated meconium consists of initial depression, labored respirations and tachypnea. Chest x-ray shows bilateral coarse infiltrates with spots of hyperaeration, producing a honeycomb effect. The infant is treated with oxygen for cyanosis and with antibiotics (e.g., penicillin and kanamycin); the latter are required because the differentiation of meconium aspiration and bacterial pneumonia is difficult and because meconium aspiration may predispose to bacterial pneumonia.

Pneumonia

Pneumonia may be acquired prenatally, intranatally or postnatally. Onset of symptoms occurs at birth in the infant infected in utero and somewhat later in the infant infected at birth or shortly thereafter.

Factors predisposing to intrauterine infection include prolonged rupture of membranes (greater than 24 hours), prolonged labor (with or without ruptured membranes) and increased obstetric manipulation. Placental, skin and gastric aspirate cultures should be obtained whenever such a history is given.

The infant may have delayed respirations at birth, dyspnea, tachypnea, retractions and cyanosis. Irregular respirations may be noted, with apneic episodes. Fever is more common in the term infant, whereas hypothermia is seen in the premature. Chest x-rays show poorly defined, streaky densities which are occasionally unilateral. Air bronchograms are seen because of exudate-filled alveoli adjacent to air-filled bronchi, and the cardiac borders may be indistinct because of adjacent infiltrates.

Cultures of blood, throat and tracheal aspirate should be obtained, followed by immediate institution of antibiotic therapy. General supportive care is given as described above for hyaline membrane disease.

Pulmonary Hemorrhage

The infant with pulmonary hemorrhage presents clinically like one with hyaline membrane disease, showing tachypnea, retractions and cyanosis. Bleeding from the upper airway is seen in approximately 50% of cases. Chest x-ray usually shows nonspecific changes: a reticulogranular appearance, nodular densities, opacification and normal appearance have been described.

Treatment consists in transfusion of fresh heparinized blood, administration of oxygen, and general supportive measures. If there is evidence of disseminated intravascular coagulation, heparinization is indicated. The prognosis is extremely poor.

Anatomic Pulmonary Disorders

Pulmonary agenesis and hypoplasia. Unilateral pulmonary agenesis occurs more frequently than bilateral agenesis and may be familial, whereas the latter is not. The left lung is more frequently involved, with compensatory enlargement of the remaining lung, which may herniate into the involved side of the chest. There is a marked deviation of the trachea, and the mediastinal contents are displaced. Externally, the chest may appear symmetrical.

Pulmonary hypoplasia often occurs with other malformations, notably diaphragmatic hernia and renal agenesis (Potter's syndrome). Right-to-left shunting through a perfused but nonventilated hypoplastic lung may be relieved by resection of the involved lung.

Lobar emphysema. The infant with congenital lobar emphysema may have respiratory distress shortly after birth, although the more common occurrence is for respiratory distress to follow infection at 1-2 months of age. Retractions, cyanosis and wheezing may be noted, with the severity of symptoms paralleling the degree of involvement. Chest x-ray shows a radiolucent lobe; the mediastinum may be shifted to the uninvolved side when overdistention is severe. The diagnosis may be confused with that of pulmonary cyst unless lung markings can be identified in the radiolucency.

Bronchoscopy should be done, because occasionally an obstruction will be found and its removal will alleviate symptoms immediately. More often lobectomy is necessary. The asymptomatic infant may be treated conservatively after bronchoscopy, inasmuch as recovery may occur without lobectomy in such infants.

Pulmonary cysts. Congenital lung cysts may occur either in the periphery of the lung or centrally (bronchogenic cysts). Peripheral cysts may lack a communication with bronchi. They may be multiple and present a honeycomb appearance on x-ray rather than the single radiolucent area of one cyst. The trachea may be shifted to the uninvolved side. Bronchogenic cysts may present with episodes of stridor, wheezing and infection rather than respiratory distress in the first hours of life. They may obstruct a bronchus and result in atelectasis or overdistention. Bronchograms may demonstrate the cyst or bronchial compression, depending on whether the cyst communicates with the bronchus or obstructs it.

Resection should be done without delay in the symptomatic infant. It should probably be done in the asymptomatic infant, because of compression of normal lung and the risk of infection.

Pulmonary adenomatoid malformation. This disorder consists of a collection of cysts in any part of the lung, with polypoid epithelial proliferation. The infant is often prematurely born and has respiratory distress shortly after birth. Chest x-rays show a mass with scattered areas of radiolucency; there may be mediastinal shift and large cystic areas. Treatment consists in lobectomy, in symptomatic infants.

Accessory and sequestered lobes. These are usually not symptomatic in the newborn period but may be mistaken for other lesions: they appear as radiopaque chest masses. Accessory lobes are separate from the remainder of the lung; sequestered lobes are parts of lung which do not have the normal relationship to the rest of the pulmonary tissue. The usual sequestered lobe is seen to be surrounded by normal lower lobe, and its vascular supply is directly from the aorta.

Pulmonary lymphangiectasis. Dilatation of pulmonary lymphatics may occur alone or may be associated with intestinal lymphangiectasia. Other anomalies—notably congenital heart disease—may coexist. Respiratory distress usually occurs at birth or shortly thereafter. Chest x-ray shows hyperaeration and resembles that of hyaline membrane disease.

Diaphragmatic Disorders

Paralysis. Phrenic nerve paralysis results from trauma at delivery and is usually associated with brachial paralysis. Lateral hyperextension of the neck can result in injury to the brachial plexus and the anterior roots of the phrenic nerve; infants with difficult breech extractions and shoulder dystocia are most at risk. The diagnosis can be suspected in such an infant when there is unilateral absence of arm movement (easily demonstrated by eliciting a Moro reflex) associated with tachypnea. X-ray shows slight elevation of the diaphragm on the affected side initially; this becomes more pronounced later. Fluoroscopy shows normal diaphragmatic motion on the unaffected side; the affected side shows a paradoxical rise with inspiration and descent with expiration. Atelectasis may be a persistent problem.

With mild injury, improvement is generally seen during the first week of life. Severely symptomatic infants may require plication of the diaphragm.

Eventration. Congenital muscular defects of the diaphragm result in a ballooning upward of the diaphragm on the affected side and may result in severe respiratory distress in the newborn period. Paradoxical diaphragmatic motion seen at fluoroscopy may make differentiation

from diaphragmatic paralysis impossible. If the infant is severely symptomatic and unresponsive to general supportive care, surgical plication
should be carried out.

Hernia. Diaphragmatic defects with abdominal viscera in the thoracic
cavity can cause severe respiratory difficulty. Left-sided defects are
much more common than right-sided ones. The heart is usually displaced to the uninvolved side, and bowel sounds may be heard in the
chest. The abdomen is scaphoid. Bowel pattern in the chest on x-ray
may occasionally be confused with cystic disease of the lung; typical
bowel markings may be seen, however.

Treatment consists in immediate surgical repair. If it is necessary to
transport the infant to another center, this should be done with the infant in an erect position and with a nasogastric tube in place to prevent
further distention of the intrathoracic viscera with swallowed air.

Tracheoesophageal Fistula

The most common form of this disorder is esophageal atresia with a
proximal blind esophageal pouch and a connection between the trachea
and the lower esophageal pouch. Upper pouch communications and H-
type fistulas without atresia occur but are rare. Polyhydramnios is
common.

Clinically the infant presents with excessive secretions coming from
the mouth and nose, followed by aspiration pneumonia. If feeding is
attempted, the infant chokes and regurgitates immediately.

Diagnosis is made, preferably at birth and before symptoms appear,
by inability to pass a nasogastric tube into the stomach. A tube which
has coiled in the blind pouch can be detected by injecting a small amount
of air into the nasogastric tube while listening over the stomach with a
stethoscope. Chest x-ray shows the air-filled blind pouch. Air in the
stomach and small bowel indicates that the trachea communicates with
the lower pouch. It is only rarely necessary to instill contrast material
for visualization of the upper pouch; use of a radiopaque catheter is
usually sufficient.

Surgical correction is indicated as soon as possible after the diagnosis
is made. If it is necessary to postpone surgery because of severe pneumonia, a suction catheter in the pouch is essential.

Intrathoracic Cysts and Tumors

Mediastinal masses may present with tachypnea, dyspnea and cyanosis because of compression of the trachea or bronchi. The radiographic appearance of different types of tumors and cysts may be similar, and differentiation may be possible only by surgical exploration. Gastric cysts, neuroblastomas, neurofibromas and ganglioneuromas are most commonly seen in the posterior mediastinum, whereas teratomas are more frequently anterior in position. Cystic hygromas may extend into the superior mediastinum.

Pneumothorax and Pneumomediastinum

Rupture of alveoli with entry of air into the pleural space or mediastinum can occur spontaneously or as the result of overzealous resuscitation. If symptomatic, the infant shows tachypnea, grunting, retractions and cyanosis. The severity of symptoms depends on the amount of air present. Irritability and restlessness are common. Sudden deterioration in an improving infant with hyaline membrane disease should always suggest the presence of a pneumothorax. Isolated pneumomediastinum may be asymptomatic.

In unilateral pneumothorax, the physical examination shows displacement of the apical cardiac impulse; the involved side of the chest may appear prominent. It may be possible to detect a decrease of breath sounds. Chest x-ray shows a peripheral radiolucency in which lung markings are absent. The lung can be visualized centrally and may show varying degrees of collapse. In pneumomediastinum a halo of air surrounds the heart and the thymus is lifted up to produce the so-called sail sign; lateral views show air between the anterior cardiac border and the sternum.

Spontaneous improvement may occur; or the pneumothorax may require needle aspiration. Breathing of 100% oxygen hastens resorption of a pneumothorax. Sudden change in vital signs indicates air under tension; for the infant with known pneumothorax, equipment for emergency aspiration (18-gauge needle, three-way stopcock and 50-ml. syringe) should be immediately available. With continued air leak, it may be necessary to insert a chest tube for continuous water-seal drainage.

Pleural Effusion; Chylothorax

This rare disorder presents with tachypnea, retractions and cyanosis, usually shortly after birth. When unilateral, there is displacement of the midline structures away from the effusion; decreased breath sounds and dullness may be present. Bilateral effusion is rare.

Chest x-ray reveals opacification of the involved hemithorax. Thoracentesis yields clear pleural fluid unless oral milk feedings have been given; the fluid becomes opalescent after the institution of fat-containing formula.

Treatment consists in repeated thoracenteses. Most cases resolve after one or more taps. In resistant cases (no improvement after 6-8 weeks of repeated removal of fluid) surgical exploration should be carried out. Repairable leakage of the thoracic duct may be demonstrated. Feeding of medium-chain triglycerides (which enter the portal system rather than the lymphatic system) may be useful.

Transient Tachypnea of the Newborn

This syndrome, first described by Avery et al. in 1966, is marked by increased respiratory rates (to 120/minute) without retractions in newborn infants who do not otherwise appear ill. Chest x-ray shows prominent streaking in the hilar areas; this condition is believed to represent delayed resorption of fetal lung fluid, with resultant dilatation of the perivascular lymphatics. Symptoms improve spontaneously.

Wilson-Mikity Syndrome

This disorder of the prematurely born infant is characterized by cyanosis, normal or increased respiratory rates, and a roentgenographic picture of multiple cyst-like foci of hyperaeration, producing the "bubbly lung" appearance. Symptoms may appear at birth or as late as 1 month of age. The usual onset of symptoms is just after the first week of life; symptoms become most severe 4-8 weeks later and improve slowly thereafter. The course is prolonged—increased environmental oxygen may be needed for as long as 6 months—but complete recovery is possible.

SUGGESTED READINGS

1. Avery, M. E., Gatewood, O. B., and Brumley, G.: Transient tachypnea of the newborn, Am. J. Dis. Child. 111:380, 1966.
2. Behrman, R. E.: The use of acid-base measurements in the clinical evaluation and treatment of the sick neonate, J. Pediat. 74:632, 1969.
3. Chu, J., et al.: Preliminary report: The pulmonary hypoperfusion syndrome, Pediatrics 35:733, 1965.
4. Harrison, V. C., Heese, H. de V., and Klein, M.: The significance of grunting in hyaline membrane disease, Pediatrics 41:549, 1968.
5. Hey, E. N., and Katz, G.: The optimum thermal environment for naked babies, Arch. Dis. Childhood 45:328, 1970.
6. Nelson, N. M.: On the etiology of hyaline membrane disease, Pediat. Clin. North America 17:943, 1970.
7. Strauss, J.: Tris(hydroxymethyl)amino-methane (THAM): A pediatric evaluation, Pediatrics 41:667, 1968.

CHAPTER 6

Hyperbilirubinemia

YOSHIO MIYAZAKI, M.D.
G. VAN LEEUWEN, M.D.

Since about 1948, pediatricians have accepted the use of exchange transfusion in infants with hemolytic disease of the newborn due to Rh and ABO incompatibility whose indirect bilirubin approached or exceeded 20 mg./100 ml. It was well documented and accepted that indirect bilirubin levels exceeding 20 mg./100 ml. were associated with a high incidence of kernicterus in the infant.

Only in the last few years have we become convinced that lower levels of bilirubin are dangerous as well, particularly for the distressed infant or the infant of less than 38 weeks' gestational age. There is now reasonable evidence that infants of low birthweight have an increasingly high incidence of mental and motor retardation associated with high levels of total serum bilirubin (Fig. 6-1). In a study by Boggs, Fardy and Frazier, 23,000 infants were observed from birth. Tests of mental and motor development were administered by a psychologist to these infants at age eight months. The findings suggested a positive relationship between increasing neonatal hyperbilirubinemia and the incidence of low mental or motor scores at age eight months. These relationships did not begin abruptly at the level of 20 mg./100 ml.; rather, they rose progressively and became substantial at the level of 16-19 mg./100 ml.

Stern and co-workers have found definite histologic evidence of kernicterus in small infants with fatal outcome from hyaline membrane syndrome who in some instances had serum indirect bilirubin levels as low as 12 mg./100 ml.

It appears, then, that there is a major risk, particularly to the small or distressed baby, if serum indirect bilirubin levels are much in excess of 10 mg./100 ml. In such cases, the major objective of therapy is to keep the serum indirect bilirubin below 12-14 mg./100 ml. How various thera-

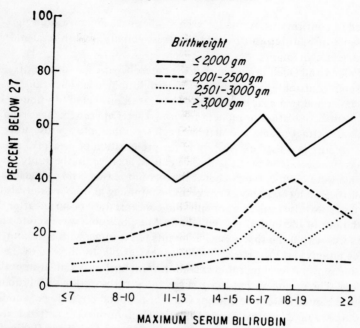

Fig. 6-1.—Percentage of total motor scores below 27. (From Boggs, T. R., Fardy, J. B., and Frazier, T. M.: Correlation of neonatal serum total bilirubin concentrations and developmental status at age eight months, J. Pediat. 71:553, 1967.)

peutic approaches have been developed, their pharmacologic action and their possible untoward effects will be described. The three therapeutic agents to be discussed are blue light, alcohol and phenobarbital. We will conclude with recommendations for the treatment of hyperbilirubinemia **not** due to Rh or ABO incompatibility.

ETIOLOGY OF NONHEMOLYTIC HYPERBILIRUBINEMIA

Immaturity of liver function—specifically, decreased glucuronyl transferase activity—has been indicated as the prime cause of "physiologic jaundice" and an increase of bilirubin production as a secondary contributor to hyperbilirubinemia. However, a number of studies have failed to confirm this. Actually, some studies have demonstrated the presence of bilirubin glucuronyl transferase activity in both fetal and normal human infants.

Poland and Odell proposed that the enterohepatic circulation of bilirubin contributes to physiologic hyperbilirubinemia. These authors demonstrated that agar in a thioglycolate broth protected bilirubin from either oxidation or reduction during bacterial growth. Agar is an aqueous extract of seaweed that has been separated into agarose and agaropectin. It is used extensively in the preservation of meat, fish, etc. It has also been used medicinally as a colloid laxative. In the study, the infants were given 250 mg. of agar powder in the first 5 ml. of each formula, beginning at 20 hours of age and continuing at 4-hour intervals for 24 doses. No rise in the serum bilirubin concentration occurred after the 13th hour of life in the agar-fed infants. More bilirubin was excreted in the feces within the first 5 days in infants fed formula with agar, and these infants also lost less weight than the controls. By the end of the sixth day, total fecal bilirubin excretion from birth was similar in both groups. The results of that study suggest that reabsorption of bilirubin from the intestine can be a major cause of neonatal physiologic jaundice. Certainly a mild laxative given to the small infant or the infant at risk would be preferable to any other therapeutic modality, if the findings of these two investigators are confirmed.

In summary: the increased bilirubin is not, for the most part, due to excessive hemolysis. Hyperbilirubinemia of this type may be partly due to immaturity of the liver and glucuronyl transferase deficiency, but may well be primarily due to reabsorption of bilirubin already present in the intestinal tract at birth.

PHOTOTHERAPY

The effectiveness of phototherapy with blue fluorescent light to prevent hyperbilirubinemia of prematurity was clearly documented by Lucey and co-workers in 1968 (Fig. 6-2). Ten years earlier, Cremer et al. had demonstrated that serum bilirubin concentrations of some infants could be reduced by exposure to sunlight or artificial blue light. Several other groups (English, South American, French and Italian) also reported satisfactory experiences with light therapy.

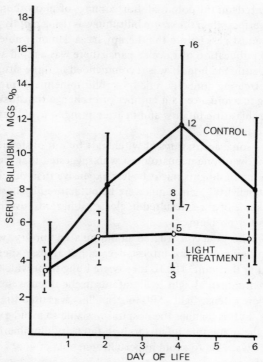

Fig. 6-2.—Prevention of hyperbilirubinemia of prematurity by phototherapy. (From Lucey, J., Ferreiro, M., and Hewitt, J.: Prevention of hyperbilirubinemia of prematurity by phototherapy, Pediatrics 41:1047, 1968.)

As initially described, this form of therapy was intended to prevent the jaundice common to low-birthweight infants and believed due primarily to glucuronyl transferase deficiency. That this could be done was clearly demonstrated by Lucey. Each infant in the light-treated group was placed under ten 20-watt bulbs during the first 12 hours of life and was exposed continuously until 144 hours of age.

Early experience suggested the possibility of retinal damage from this much light. (The original study group did have eye protection.) Damage to the rods and cones in as short a period as 12 hours has been documented in prematurely born kittens.

Lucey pointed out the potential shortcomings of phototherapy: (1) there was less effect when the serum bilirubin was rising rapidly and (2) several hours must pass before the therapy has a demonstrable effect.

Following publication of Lucey's paper there was a rapid acceptance of this therapeutic method. It was recommended in three situations primarily: in treating nonhemolytic hyperbilirubinemia of prematurity; in attempting to avoid a certain number of exchange transfusions in mildly erythroblastotic infants; and in attempting to avoid some repeat exchange transfusions.

There were some accusations of witchcraft by our obstetric colleagues. We know of one neonatologist who suggested that medical students holding flashlights might be less expensive than purchasing the $500 "bilirubin light." Many units were manufactured by hospital electricians; some of these resulted in electrical hazards, overheated babies, and other problems.

At least one hospital constructed an illuminated nursery, which delivered phototherapy to a less intense degree, but at less expense, to all babies placed in that unit. The fixtures were hung to provide 90 footcandles of environmental light to all infants in the intensive-care nursery. A more intense light—500 footcandles—was used for the jaundiced infants. In this manner the hospital was able to avoid exposing over 80% of the premature infants to high-intensity illumination and at the same time was able to avoid hyperbilirubinemia in 96.9% of the premature infants.

The biochemical change effected by phototherapy has not been totally elucidated. Callahan and co-workers, using tracer amounts of ^{14}C-bilirubin in two infants with Crigler-Najjar syndrome, were able to make some observations. They showed that light converts bilirubin in vivo to more polar, predominantly diazo-negative and presumably less toxic derivatives, which were rapidly excreted in bile and urine without detectable plasma retention.

Concepts change rapidly after a new therapeutic regimen is described. This has been true of phototherapy for hyperbilirubinemia. After a number of modifications, Behrman and Hsia have summarized the current status of phototherapy, with which we basically agree. One clear hazard of phototherapy is retinal damage; therefore, nursery personnel must be watchful of total eye-covering at all times. There is a suspicion but no absolute evidence at this time that phototherapy may be associated with retardation in weight, length and head circumference.

Phototherapy has some usefulness, then, in the small or distressed infant with serum indirect bilirubin levels of 10-15 mg./100 ml. There may be some benefit in reducing the need for exchange transfusion and in preventing brain injury in term infants with hemolytic disease or septicemia, but there is no evidence for this. **Phototherapy should not be used prophylactically at this time.** Specific recommendations are given at the conclusion of this chapter.

ALCOHOL

There have been reports that after alcohol (ethanol) has been administered intravenously to mothers in premature labor, in an attempt to arrest labor, their infants have had significantly less jaundice.

We have had limited experience with infants born under these circumstances, but we have encountered two who seemed to be profoundly inebriated, and in whom we had to provide ventilatory assistance for several hours before they recovered.

We do not recommend at this time that alcohol be considered seriously as a drug for preventing neonatal hyperbilirubinemia.

PHENOBARBITAL

Phenobarbital has been clearly shown to reduce the concentration of total serum bilirubin in the neonate—most effectively if given to the mother during the last stages of pregnancy but also if given to the infant in a dose range of 5-10 mg./kg. per day. When given to the infant the drug is apparently less effective if initiated after jaundice has appeared.

Pharmacologically the drug appears to work at many levels to accelerate bilirubin transport. There is definitely an increase in liver glucuronyl transferase activity. There may be an increase in Y protein of the liver and increased bilirubin uptake by the liver cell. It is also known that phenobarbital enhances some of the metabolic activities of the membranes of the endoplasmic reticulum, including bilirubin glucuronide formation.

As with phototherapy, there is ample evidence that this drug can both prevent and treat elevated serum bilirubin. Untoward effects, if any, of this method of treatment are as yet essentially unknown, at least in humans. Until a lack of untoward effects is certain, we hesitate to recommend phenobarbital except in properly designed experimental studies.

A number of known and postulated side effects of phenobarbital warrant the caution expressed above. Among these are (1) stimulation of liver microsomal enzymes that metabolize steroid hormones and (2) delayed effects of barbiturates on later sexual development and behavior. However, no evidence exists to date that the human infant is harmed by phenobarbital. There is a known effect of phenobarbital on the clotting mechanism; but Doxiadis encountered no bleeding or hemorrhagic episodes in his infants. Whatever problems might arise could presumably be prevented by giving vitamin K to the mother concomitantly with the phenobarbital or, as is already standard practice, administering natural vitamin K to the newborn.

Doxiadis concluded that phenobarbital administered during the last stages of pregnancy reduces both the absolute level and the duration of neonatal jaundice. However, nothing is known as to possible long-term endocrine or other effects.

The physician must use his clinical judgment as to whether he will prescribe phenobarbital for certain pregnant women. Should he give it to women whose previous infants have had icterus? To those entering premature labor? To those who have previously given birth to a risk infant? He may, of course, elect to treat the baby after birth. Perhaps is is wiser to await further information here also.

DIAGNOSIS AND TREATMENT OF HYPERBILIRUBINEMIA

Diagnosis. All infants—term or preterm, well or sick—should have at least one serum bilirubin determination if they appear jaundiced. A new instrument, called a bilirubinometer, is ideal for this purpose. A total serum bilirubin can be done with two drops of serum, and the results are within 5-10% of those obtained in the central laboratory. The procedure is easily done by the nursing personnel. The machine measures only total bilirubin, so it cannot be used when the level exceeds 15 mg./100 ml.; i.e., when the level of serum indirect bilirubin becomes critical.

If the bilirubin exceeds 10 mg./100 ml. repeat determinations should be performed at intervals of 4-12 hours until a falling bilirubin level is documented. This is important, not only to the baby but also for medicolegal reasons.

Treatment. Treatment suggested below is based on present knowledge and may change rapidly. Bear in mind that bilirubin levels, here, refer to serum **indirect** bilirubin. The treatment described generally applies to babies who do not have hemolytic disease, but there is overlapping. It should be noted that fresh (less than day-old) adult blood contains 2,3-diphosphoglycerate, which has the ability to release oxygen to the tissues; therefore, adult blood as fresh as possible should always be used when blood is given, for any reason, to a sick baby.

In infants with hyperbilirubinemia—particularly those at risk—the total serum protein should be kept greater than 5.0 Gm./100 ml. because of the albumin-bilirubin binding. As long as free albumin is present to bind bilirubin, the likelihood of kernicterus is decreased. Serum protein analysis can be very easily performed with a refractometer costing as little as $150. We believe that the more critically ill the infant is for other reasons, the more critical it becomes to maintain the serum proteins in excess of 5.0 Gm./100 ml. Human serum albumin in doses of 4 ml./kg. can safely be given intravenously slowly without danger of producing hypervolemic shock.

Treatment of choice may be summarized as follows:

Term, Well Infant

1. Bilirubin level less than 10 mg./100 ml.: no cause for concern.
2. Bilirubin 10-15 mg./100 ml.: repeat determinations frequently.
3. Bilirubin 15-20 mg./100 ml.: use phototherapy.
4. Bilirubin in excess of 20 mg./100 ml.: perform exchange transfusion if the baby is less than 96 hours old. If the baby is more than 96 hours old you may wait until the bilirubin level has reached 25 mg./100 ml.

Sick, Small (2,500-Gm.) or Risk Infant

1. Bilirubin level less than 10 mg./100 ml.: observe and repeat determinations.
2. Bilirubin 10-15 mg./100 ml.: use phototherapy.
3. Bilirubin in excess of 15 mg./100 ml.: perform exchange transfusion.

New nurseries under construction should have facilities providing 100 footcandles of light continuously; but include plans to double this if needed.

Some possible alternatives, which we do not advise at the present time, would be to (1) prevent jaundice in the risk infant either by administering phenobarbital to the mother in the late stages of pregnancy or to the baby in a dose of 5-10 mg./kg. per day and (2) use phenobarbital in a dose of 5-10 mg./kg. per day to treat jaundice when it develops.

We confess to some bias toward a rather frequent resorting to exchange transfusion in these situations. At least the results are predictable, the long-term effects are known, and the risk in experienced hands is minimal.

SUGGESTED READINGS

1. Behrman, R. E.: Phototherapy and hyperbilirubinemia, J. Pediat. 74:989, 1969.
2. Boggs, T. R., Fardy, J. B., and Frazier, T. M.: Correlation of neonatal serum total bilirubin concentrations and developmental status at age eight months, J. Pediat. 71:553, 1967.
3. Callahan, E. W., Thaler, M., Karon, M., Bauer, K., and Schmid, R.: Phototherapy of severe unconjugated hyperbilirubinemia: Formation and removal of labeled bilirubin derivatives, Pediatrics 46:841, 1970.
4. Cremer, R. J., Perryman, P. W., and Richard, D. H.: Influence of light on the hyperbilirubinemia of infants, Lancet 1:1094, 1958.
5. Franklin, A. W.: Influence of light on the hyperbilirubinemia of infants, Lancet 1:1227, 1958.
6. Guinta, F.: A one-year experience with phototherapy for jaundice of prematurity, Pediatrics 47:123, 1971.
7. Lucey, J. F.: Hyperbilirubinemia of prematurity, Pediatrics 25:690, 1960.
8. Lucey, J., Ferreiro, M., and Hewitt, J.: Prevention of hyperbilirubinemia of prematurity by phototherapy, Pediatrics 41:1047, 1968.
9. Maurer, H. M., Wolff, J. A., Poppers, P. J., Kuntzman, R., Finster, M., Pantruck, E., and Conney, A. H.: Reduction in concentration of total serum bilirubin in offspring of women treated with phenobarbitone during pregnancy, Lancet 11:122, 1968.
10. Poland, R., and Odell, G.: Physiologic jaundice: The enterohepatic circulation of bilirubin, New England J. Med. 284:1, 1971.

11. Sisson, T. R. C., Glauser, S. C., Glauser, E. M., Tasman, W., and
Kuwabara, T.: Retinal changes produced by phototherapy, J.
Pediat. 77:221, 1970.

12. Trolle, D.: Decrease of total serum bilirubin concentration in newborn infants after phenobarbitone treatment, Lancet 11:705,
1968.

13. Valaes, R., Petmezake, S., and Doxiadis, S. A.: The Effect on
Neonatal Hyperbilirubinemia of Phenobarbital during Pregnancy
or after Birth, in Bergsma, D. (ed.): *Bilirubin Metabolism in the
Newborn,* National Foundation, Birth Defects Orig. Art. Ser.
6:46, 1970.

14. Walker, W., Hughes, M. I., and Barton, M.: Barbiturate and hyperbilirubinemia of prematurity, Lancet 1:548, 1969.

CHAPTER 7

Hemolytic Disease, Anemia and Hemorrhagic Disorders

JOHN N. LUKENS, M.D.

The cellular composition and the physiologic efficiency of the blood of the neonate are characterized by rapid change. The uniqueness of hematopoiesis at this time in life is related in part to a shift in the type of hemoglobin which is synthesized, in part to the sudden transition from the relative hypoxia of intrauterine life to an oxygen-rich environment, and in part to the sequelae of fetal-maternal interactions. Recognition and proper management of hematologic disorders of the newborn necessitate familiarity with the peculiarities which characterize blood at the time of birth. For this reason, the hematologic profile of the normal neonate will be described before specific hematologic disorders are discussed.

HEMATOLOGIC PROFILE OF THE NORMAL NEONATE

Erythropoiesis in late fetal life may be likened to that of the adult· at a high altitude. In response to the hypoxic stimulus of reduced atmospheric pressure, the elaboration of erythrocyte-stimulating hormone (erythropoietin) is increased. This, in turn, is responsible for an expansion of the erythroid marrow, an increased delivery of young red blood cells to the peripheral blood and an elevation of the hemoglobin concentration. In the same fashion, the peripheral blood of the normal neonate is characterized by erythrocytosis, reticulocytosis and normoblastosis (Table 7-1). Red blood cells produced by a stimulated marrow are larger than normal (macrocytes) and experience a shortened survival (stress reticulocytes). As a result the mean corpuscular volume (MCV) of cord erythrocytes is increased and the survival of the neonate's red cells is only about two-thirds that of the adult's red cells.

With birth the hypoxic stimulus of intrauterine life is removed. Serum erythropoietin falls abruptly to an undetectable level, thereby "turning off" the erythroid marrow. During the first week of life nucleated erythrocytes disappear from the peripheral blood and reticulocytes decrease in number. Despite the postnatal arrest of erythropoiesis, an increase in the venous hemoglobin is observed during the first day of life. This increase results in part from transfusion of placental blood at birth and in part from a shift of fluid from intravascular to extravascular spaces. By 7-10 days of age the hemoglobin has returned to the level observed in cord blood. Thereafter the hemoglobin concentration drifts slowly downward until 6-8 weeks of age. A decrease in hemoglobin during the first week to a level less than that of cord blood is indicative of blood loss or hemolysis.

Normal Values

The values summarized in Table 7-1 represent smoothed means and 95% confidence limits of data taken from a number of published studies (Guest et al.; Oski and Naiman). Proper interpretation of hematologic data requires knowledge of the source from which the sample was obtained. The packed cell volume (hematocrit) of capillary blood is approximately 6% higher than that of venous blood. The hemoglobin concentration of arterial blood averages 0.5 Gm./100 ml. higher than that of venous blood.

The values for hemoglobin and packed cell volume of blood from prematurely born infants are similar to those for term infants. The numbers of reticulocytes and nucleated erythrocytes, however, are greater in the premature infant. Cord blood of infants born at 30-36 weeks' gestation contains 6-10% reticulocytes. As in term infants, an abrupt decrease in reticulocytes is observed after the third day of life. An average of 21 nucleated red blood cells per 100 white blood cells is reported in the cord blood of premature infants. Although red cell nuclei are rapidly cleared from the circulation, an occasional nucleated erythrocyte may be seen as late as 7 days of age.

Cord blood is characterized by a leukocytosis (mean white blood cells 15,000-20,000/mm.^{3}) with an absolute neutrophilia. By the third or fourth day of life the white blood cells return to 12,000/mm.^{3} or

Table 7-1. HEMATOLOGIC VALUES OF VENOUS BLOOD IN NORMAL, TERM INFANTS

Component	Cord	Day 1	Day 3	Day 7
Hgb (Gm./100 ml.)	17.0 (13.6-20.6)*	19.0 (15.0-24.0)	18.5 (14.5-23.8)	18.5 (14.5-23.8)
PCV (%)	53 (43-64)	58 (43-71)	55 (43-68)	54 (43-68)
Retic (%)	5.5 (4.2-7.2)	5.0	2.0	1.0
NRBC/100 WBC	7.3 (2.0-20.0)	3.0	0	0

Hgb = hemoglobin; PCV = packed cell volume; Retic = reticulocytes; NRBC = nucleated red blood cells
*Values represent smoothed means and 95% confidence limits

less. Of these, fewer than 50% are neutrophils. Platelets are abundant (150,000-400,000/mm.[3]). Although thrombocytopenia has been purported to be a physiologic occurrence in premature infants (Medoff), recent surveys by Fogel and others indicate that the platelet counts of thriving premature infants are no different from those of term neonates.

Red Cell 2,3-Diphosphoglycerate

In addition to its distinctive cellular composition, blood from the normal neonate differs from normal adult blood with respect to the structure of its predominant hemoglobin. An understanding of the physiologic differences between fetal hemoglobin (Hb F) and adult hemoglobin (Hb A) is of paramount importance to the physician involved with the care of sick infants.

The surrender of oxygen to tissue by Hb A is facilitated by red cell 2,3-diphosphoglycerate (2,3-DPG). This intermediate of anaerobic glycolysis combines reversibly with oxyhemoglobin to decrease the affinity of hemoglobin for oxygen: $HbO_2 + 2,3\text{-}DPG \rightleftharpoons HbDPG + O_2$. As the level of red cell 2,3-DPG increases, the affinity of the hemoglobin molecule for oxygen decreases. As a result, oxygen is unloaded from red cells to tissues at higher tissue oxygen tensions. Conversely, a decrease in red cell 2,3-DPG is associated with an increase in the affinity of hemoglobin for oxygen. With low levels of red cell 2,3-DPG, tissue hypoxia may be observed despite good blood oxygenation.

Fetal hemoglobin does not interact with 2,3-DPG to the same extent as Hb A. Although the level of red cell 2,3-DPG in cord blood is similar to that found in blood from older children and adults, its physiologic activity is limited by the concentration of Hb A. Inasmuch as Hb F accounts for 50-85% of the hemoglobin in cord blood, the "functional" DPG of normal cord blood is only 15-50% that of adult blood (Oski et al., 1970). The efficiency of tissue respiration in the newborn is further compromised by illness. Decreased levels of red cell 2,3-DPG are observed in infants with respiratory distress syndrome and in infants with sepsis. As a result, the "functional" DPG of blood from the sick neonate may be only one-sixth that of adult blood. An increase in the oxygen affinity of hemoglobin, superimposed on a decrease in arterial oxy-

110 A Manual of Newborn Medicine

gen tension, creates severe tissue hypoxia. Fortunately, both red cell 2,3-DPG and the proportion of Hb A may be increased by the transfusion of fresh adult red cells. The "functional" DPG of the neonate is increased to that of a 6-month-old by a simple exchange transfusion. For this reason, an exchange transfusion should be considered in any infant with severe cardiorespiratory insufficiency.

The discussion which follows is designed to review those hematologic states which are of particular practical or numerical significance. The reader is referred to the treatise by Oski and Naiman (see Suggested Readings) for a comprehensive analysis of hematologic disorders of the newborn.

NEONATAL ANEMIAS

Anemia in the first weeks of life may be defined as a venous hemoglobin of less than 13.5 Gm/100 ml. or a venous packed cell volume of less than 45%. The diagnostic considerations prompted by the anemic neonate are different from those invoked to explain anemia in the older infant and child. Iron deficiency, the most prevalent cause of anemia in the pediatric age group after 6 months of age, is rarely seen in the neonatal period. Although the causes of neonatal anemia are legion, the more commonly encountered anemias are relatively few. These are conveniently classified on the basis of the age at which anemia is detected (Table 7-2).

Erythroblastosis Fetalis

Isoimmune hemolytic disease continues to be the most common hematologic condition requiring therapy in the neonatal period. In the discussion which follows, primary consideration will be given to the diagnosis and postnatal management of the infant with erythroblastosis fetalis. The interested reader will find in the recent literature comprehensive reviews of the subject (Allen and Diamond) as well as detailed instruction in the technic of exchange transfusion (Bowman et al., 1970; Mauer; Pochedly), recommendations for the prenatal management of the sensitized fetus (Oski and Naiman; Bowman et al., 1969), and experience to date with the prevention of Rhesus immunization (Pollack et al.).

Table 7-2. ANEMIAS OF THE NEWBORN

Anemia present at birth

    Erythroblastosis fetalis
    Blood loss anemia

Anemia with onset after first day of life

    Blood loss
    Infection
    Hereditary spherocytosis
    Congenital nonspherocytic hemolytic anemias

Pathogenesis. Most, if not all, pregnancies are associated with the leakage of fetal erythrocytes into the maternal circulation. Although small fetal-maternal transfusions may be documented in the second and third trimesters, most transplacental hemorrhages are thought to occur during delivery of the fetus and separation of the placenta. The risk of fetal isoimmunization is determined by the antigenicity of those red cell antigens not shared by the mother and by the type of maternal antibody directed against fetal antigens. Of the many red cell antigens which have been implicated in the pathogenesis of erythroblastosis fetalis, A, B and D are of greatest clinical significance. In addition to D, other Rh antigens (C, c, E, e) may be responsible for erythroblastosis. These and "minor" blood group factors are implicated in only about 2% of infants with erythroblastosis.

Antibodies to red cell antigens are of two types. Those antibodies directed against Rh antigens are designated "immune" or "acquired." In contrast, the production of antibodies to A and B substances does not require exposure to A and B antigens. Anti-A and anti-B are naturally occurring antibodies which are present from birth in those persons whose red cells lack these antigens. "Natural" antibodies are predominantly of the IgM class of immunoglobulins. Because of their size, they do not traverse the placenta. Acquired antibodies, on the other hand, belong to the IgG class of immunoglobulins. These 7-S gamma globulins are transported across the placenta by an active metabolic process and attach themselves to antigenic sites on fetal red cells. Erythrocytes thus sensitized are removed from the circulation by fetal reticuloendothelial cells. Because the bilirubin derived from heme catabolism is readily cleared by the placenta, hemolysis is not paralleled by hyperbilirubinemia during fetal life. In response to shortened red cell survival, fetal erythropoietic effort is expanded and accelerated. To the extent that exaggerated red cell destruction is not compensated by accelerated production, the hemoglobin concentration falls. Severe fetal anemia may precipitate congestive heart failure, generalized anasarca and intrauterine death.

Because antibodies against A and B antigens are predominantly of the naturally occurring IgM type, red cell sensitization due to anti-A or anti-B is an infrequent complication of ABO-incompatible pregnancies. When encountered, ABO incompatibility is seen almost exclusively in the offspring of group-O mothers. This appears to be due to the fact that a portion of the isohemagglutinins (anti-A and anti-B) in group-O individuals is "immune" IgG. In contrast, the isohemagglutinins of persons of groups A and B are almost entirely of the IgM class. It follows that exposure to A antigen is not a prerequisite for "immune" anti-A synthesis in group-O individuals. For this reason, neonatal hemolytic disease due to AO or BO incompatibility is encountered in the offspring of first pregnancies. On the other hand, isoimmune hemolytic disease due to Rh (D) incompatibility is observed almost exclusively in the infants of mothers who have been sensitized by previous pregnancies or by previous incompatible blood transfusion.

Clinical features. The clinical expression of erythroblastosis is determined by the severity of the hemolytic process and by the maturity of the infant at birth. Severe erythrocyte sensitization is associated with pronounced anemia. Anemia, in turn, may be attended by all the complications of chronic circulatory overload: generalized anasarca, enlargement of liver and spleen, and congestive heart failure (hydrops fetalis). For reasons which are not clear, thrombocytopenic purpura and symptomatic hypoglycemia may complicate severe erythroblastosis. With less severe sensitization the hemolytic process is fully compensated by accelerated red cell generation. As a result, pallor is not observed. The hemolytic process is betrayed by progressive jaundice, usually within the first 24 hours of life. The magnitude of bilirubinemia is determined by by the load of bilirubin transported to the liver relative to hepatic conjugating capacity. Rapid increases in serum bilirubin can be anticipated in sensitized premature infants. Most of the serum bilirubin is unconjugated ("indirect") bilirubin. In severely affected infants an increase in conjugated ("direct") bilirubin is also observed.

In approximately 4% of infants with isoimmune hemolytic disease due to Rh (D) incompatibility, the hemolytic process is so mild that neither jaundice nor anemia poses a problem during the immediate neonatal period. Nevertheless, subclinical hemolysis continues into the second month of life. Because the erythroid marrow during the first 6 weeks is relatively insensitive to the stress of anemia, shortened survival of red cells is not compensated by increased production, and this gives rise to a severe "late" anemia. For this reason serial blood counts should be obtained during the first 6 weeks of life from all infants with hemolytic disease.

Isoimmunization due to ABO incompatibility is rarely associated with anemia at birth. Jaundice, the sole clinical expression of hemolysis, is often detected in the first 24 hours of life. Thereafter it progresses in intensity until the third or fourth day. In 8-10% of affected infants the magnitude of hyperbilirubinemia is sufficient to require one or more exchange transfusions. Clinically apparent ABO incompatibility is rarely encountered in the premature infant. It has been suggested that the fetus and the premature infant are spared because receptor sites for anti-A and anti-B globulins do not appear on red cell membranes until late in fetal life.

Hematologic features. Approximately 15% of infants with erythroblastosis due to Rh (D) incompatibility are anemic at birth (cord hemoglobin less than 13.5 Gm./100 ml.). Cord hemoglobin concentrations as low as 3-5 Gm./100 ml. have been documented in live-born infants with hydrops fetalis. During the postnatal period anemia of variable severity is seen in the vast majority of affected infants. The peripheral blood smear is characterized by normoblastosis (more than 10 nucleated red cells per 100 white blood cells) and poikilocytosis. Reticulocyte counts as high as 30% are reported.

As previously indicated, anemia at birth is not a feature of isoimmunization due to ABO incompatibility. Normoblastosis and reticulocytosis are unimpressive. The most striking feature of the peripheral blood smear is the prominence of spherocytes. Indeed, the red cell morphology and the osmotic fragility curve may be indistinguishable from those associated with hereditary spherocytosis. The two conditions are readily differentiated by the autohemolysis test.

Diagnosis. The prenatal diagnosis of erythroblastosis fetalis due to Rh (D) incompatibility may be suspected in the face of a rising anti-Rh

(D) titer (indirect Coombs test) in the mother. Because the predictive value of the antibody titer is limited, this information must be supplemented by examination of the amniotic fluid for products of heme catabolism. Serial amniocenteses permit identification of the sensitized fetus, assessment of the severity of the hemolytic process and determination of the optimal time for delivery. There is no clinically useful test for the prenatal diagnosis of isoimmunization due to ABO incompatibility.

The postnatal diagnosis of Rh (D) erythroblastosis is made by documenting Rhesus incompatibility (infant Rh (D)-positive, mother Rh (D)-negative) and detecting antibody on the infant's erythrocytes (positive direct Coombs test). Occasionally no blood group incompatibility is demonstrated in an infant with a positive direct Coombs reaction and clinically severe erythroblastosis. This perplexing situation is explained by the blocking of all available Rh (D) antigenic sites on the infant's cells by maternal antibody. As a result the infant's cells appear to be Rh (D)-negative when in fact they are Rh (D)-positive.

The diagnosis of erythroblastosis due to ABO isoimmunization rests on the demonstration of an appropriate infant-maternal incompatibility in an infant whose clinical course and hematologic features are consistent with ABO incompatibility. Ninety percent of the mothers of affected infants have group-O cells. The infant's blood type is group A or, less frequently, group B. Although red cell sensitization may be detected by a weakly positive direct Coombs test at birth, this reaction is usually negative by 24 hours of age. Conventional methods for quantitating anti-A and anti-B titers are of no diagnostic value, because they fail to distinguish 19-S (natural) from 7-S (acquired) antibodies. Unfortunately, the technics which reliably separate IgG antibodies from those of larger molecular weight are not readily adapted to the clinical laboratory. The generally available tests which purport to measure "immune" anti-A and anti-B are so crude as to render them of little practical value. Moreover, the demonstration of "immune" isohemagglutinins in maternal serum does not necessarily portend identifiable disease in the infant. Only 15% of group-A infants, born to group-O mothers whose sera contain "immune" anti-A, have laboratory or clinical evidence of hemolysis. One the other hand, failure to demonstrate immune antibodies by reliable technics excludes the diagnosis.

Treatment. The cornerstone of therapy for the infant with erythroblastosis fetalis is the exchange transfusion. This relatively crude but highly effective procedure facilitates removal of approximately 85% of sensitized red cells, reduces the serum concentration of bilirubin and permits prompt correction of congestive heart failure.

There are two clear indications for exchange transfusion in the infant with erythroblastosis: correction of anemia present at birth and maintenance of serum bilirubin below those levels which are associated with bilirubin encephalopathy. A venous hemoglobin concentration of less than 12 Gm./100 ml. at birth or during the first 24 hours of life reflects severe hemolytic disease and, as such, constitutes an indication for exchange transfusion. If untreated, infants who are anemic at birth experience a progressive decrease in hemoglobin concentration and severe hyperbilirubinemia. Congestive heart failure, the bedfellow of severe anemia, is readily corrected by exchange transfusion. By leaving a volume deficit of 10-20 ml. while increasing the circulating hemoglobin concentration, the central venous pressure may be reduced below 9 cm. of saline. Anemia which develops after the first day of life is best treated with the simple transfusion of packed cells which are compatible with the mother's blood.

The second uncontested indication for exchange transfusion is a concentration of serum bilirubin which, if not reduced, poses a risk of kernicterus. Reduction of serum bilirubin by exchange transfusion should be accomplished if (1) the serum indirect bilirubin reaches or exceeds 20 mg./100 ml.; (2) clinical manifestations of early bilirubin encephalopathy are observed; or (3) it is apparent from the rate of bilirubin rise that the peak level will exceed 20 mg./100 ml. Because otherwise healthy infants appear to be vulnerable to kernicterus only if the indirect bilirubin exceeds 20 mg./100 ml., this concentration has been accepted as the level at which exchange transfusion should be performed, irrespective of the infant's age. It is important to remember, however, that acidosis, shock, hypoxemia and a variety of drugs may displace unconjugated bilirubin from albumin, thereby predisposing to encephalopathy at bilirubin concentrations below 20 mg./100 ml. For this reason exchange transfusion should be considered for the sick neonate whose serum bilirubin is less than 20 mg./100 ml. but who demonstrates the early (and reversible) signs of bilirubin encephalopathy: lethargy, hypotonia, weak cry, poor suck and hypothermia.

Finally, because bilirubin levels in the first hours of life have predictive value with respect to the subsequent magnitude of bilirubinemia, an exchange transfusion should be performed if the bilirubin concentration exceeds 5 mg./100 ml. at birth, 10 mg./100 ml. at 8 hours, 12 mg./ 100 ml. at 16 hours or 15 mg./100 ml. at 24 hours of age.

The blood selected for exchange transfusion should be fresh (less than 3 days old) and compatible with both maternal and infant sera. Type-O, Rh (D)-negative blood is used for infants whose hemolytic disease is due to Rh (D) incompatibility; type-O, Rh (D)-compatible blood is used for infants with ABO incompatibility. It is important that a sample of the mother's blood accompany the infant who is transported from the place of birth to another institution for exchange transfusion. If severe hemolytic disease is suspected, the infant should be delivered in an institution where facilities for exchange transfusion are immediately available. For such an infant, type-O, Rh (D)-negative blood which is compatible with the mother's blood should be available in the delivery room. Although the use of citrate as an anticoagulant for donor blood has theoretical disadvantages for the neonate, acid citrate dextrose (ACD) and citrate phosphate dextrose (CPD) blood are well tolerated by mature infants. For the sick or premature infant the use of heparinized blood is preferable. A full unit of blood is used for the term infant. For low-birthweight infants the procedure is stopped after exchanging 180 ml. of blood per kilogram of body weight.

The procedure requires a skilled operator, an assistant to the operator, appropriate hardware and mechanisms for maintaining the infant's body temperature and for warming the donor blood. Instructions for performing the procedure are presented in detail elsewhere and will not be repeated here. The necessary hardware may be purchased as a disposable kit. Odell has advocated the use of an albumin infusion prior to the procedure when exchange transfusion is done for hyperbilirubinemia. The administration of 25% salt-poor human albumin (1 Gm./kg.) 1 to 2 hours prior to exchange transfusion effects a 40% increase in the bilirubin removed. Albumin priming is contraindicated in the infant with congestive heart failure. It should not be used for the initial exchange transfusion.

Although it is common practice to expose sensitized infants to artificial light, no evidence has yet been published to document the effectiveness of phototherapy in decreasing the need for exchange transfusion in infants with hemolytic disease. Because the relationship between serum bilirubin concentration and observed icterus is altered by phototherapy, it is of paramount importance that the serum bilirubin be carefully monitored if phototherapy is used.

Whether or not the infant with erythroblastosis fetalis is subjected to an exchange transfusion in the immediate neonatal period, a progressive decrease in the hemoglobin concentration during the first 6 weeks of life may be expected. This "late" anemia develops because the erythroid marrow fails to increase its production of erythrocytes in response to continuing hemolysis. A simple transfusion of sedimented red cells may be necessary if the hemoglobin falls below 5-6 Gm./100 ml. The infusion of 2 ml. of red blood cells per kilogram of body weight is followed by an increase in the hemoglobin concentration of 1 Gm./100 ml. (If whole blood is used, it is necessary to give 6 ml./kg. in order to raise the hemoglobin 1 Gm./100 ml.) Because maternal antibodies persist in the infant's circulation through the second month of life, Rh (D)-negative blood must be used. Spontaneous correction of the anemia is heralded by a reticulocytosis between 6 and 8 weeks of age.

An effective means for preventing maternal sensitization to fetal erythrocytes promises to conclude the saga of the therapeutic conquest of erythroblastosis. High-titer anti-Rh (D) antiserum (RhoGAM), given early in the postpartum period to the Rh (D)-negative mother who has delivered an Rh (D)-positive infant, effects rapid removal of fetal erythrocytes from the maternal circulation and thereby prevents maternal sensitization.

Blood Loss Anemia

Posthemorrhagic anemia in the neonate is a potentially lethal condition which, if recognized, can be effectively treated. Overt bleeding from a torn umbilicus or traumatized placenta alerts the physician to the necessity for careful surveillance of the infant's hemoglobin concentration. More commonly, however, fetal bleeding is occult and unsuspected. Leakage of fetal red cells into the maternal circulation can be documented in at least 50% of all pregnancies. Moreover, hemorrhages of significant magnitude are not uncommon. Cohen et al. estimated that 8% of apparently uncomplicated pregnancies are associated with a loss of 0.5 to 40 ml. of fetal blood into the maternal circulation. In nearly 1% of pregnancies, he calculated a delivery of 40 ml. of fetal blood to the mother. Likewise, fetal blood may escape into the circulation of a twin fetus. The ensuing erythrocytosis in the transfused fetus may be as devastating to survival as are the volume depletion and anemia in the donor twin. In addition to loss by transfusion, fetal blood may contribute to the hemorrhage associated with placenta previa and abruptio placentae or may escape into body cavities during delivery.

Clinical and hematologic features. The clinical and laboratory manifestations of posthemorrhagic anemia are determined by the volume of blood lost and by the interval of time over which the hemorrhage took place. Pallor is the most consistent feature of acute blood loss. The infant is lethargic and hypotonic. Respirations are grunting and associated with nasal flaring. The prominence of respiratory distress often lures the physician away from a consideration of the proper diagnosis. Unlike the infant whose primary problem is respiratory, the infant with acute blood loss demonstrates little or no cyanosis and fails to improve with the administration of oxygen. Capillary perfusion, as judged by the return of color to a blanched area of skin, is poor. The loss of 25-30% of the blood volume is associated with weak peripheral pulses and shock. Unlike the infant with erythroblastosis, the infant with acute blood loss has no enlargement of the liver or spleen and no increase in venous pressure.

Acute blood loss during delivery is generally not betrayed by alterations in the cord hemoglobin concentration. During the first hours of life the plasma volume expands in order to compensate for the volume deficit created by the hemorrhage. Coincident with this shift of fluid into the intravascular space, the hemoglobin concentration and packed cell volume fall. Whereas the normal infant demonstrates a rising hemoglobin concentration, the infant who has sustained a hemorrhage experiences a progressive fall in hemoglobin during the first 12 hours of life. For this reason serial counts should be done if neonatal hemorrhage is suspected.

The clinical picture of the infant who has sustained a remote or chronic blood loss is unlike that of the infant who has bled acutely. Compensatory mechanisms effect expansion of the blood volume; as a result, respiratory distress and shock are not observed. On the other hand, enlargement of the liver and spleen and an increase in the central venous pressure are the rule. As with any severe anemia, frank congestive heart failure may be present. Anicteric pallor is obvious, and the clinical impression of anemia is readily documented. The cord hemoglobin may be as low as 3 Gm./100 ml. Because the blood loss imposes a drain on fetal iron endowment, the anemia may have all the morphologic and biochemical hallmarks of iron deficiency anemia. With severe anemia peripheral blood normoblasts and reticulocytes are prominently increased.

Diagnosis. Acute natal hemorrhage is suggested by a falling hemoglobin concentration during the first hours of life. Failure to demonstrate anemia, reticulocytosis or normoblastosis in cord blood should not discourage a presumptive diagnosis. By 4-10 hours of age a drop in the hemoglobin concentration is apparent. In contrast, the infant with chronic blood loss is frankly anemic at birth and demonstrates the morphologic and biochemical features of iron deficiency. The diagnosis of both acute and chronic blood loss is reinforced by the demonstration of fetal cells in the maternal circulation. This is readily accomplished by immersing a peripheral blood smear from the mother in an acid medium for 5 minutes before staining (Kleihauer-Betke technic, described in Oski and Naiman, page 63). In an acid medium Hb A is eluted from red cells, whereas Hb F is not affected. Cells which contain Hb A appear as red cell ghosts; those which contain Hb F are normally stained. Failure to demonstrate fetal cells in maternal blood does not obviate the possibility of a fetal-maternal transfusion: fetal cells may be rapidly cleared from the maternal circulation in ABO-incompatible pregnancies. If loss of blood has been to a twin, the hemoglobin concentrations of blood from the twins should differ by more than 5 Gm./100 ml.

Acute posthemorrhagic anemia is most commonly confused with primary ventilatory problems in which asphyxia is associated with pallor rather than cyanosis (asphyxia pallida). Both conditions are characterized by pallor, respiratory distress and poor tissue perfusion. They are readily differentiated, however, by noting the heart rate and by observing the response to oxygen administration. Whereas apnea in the neonate is associated with bradycardia, posthemorrhagic hypovolemia characteristically elicits an increase in the heart rate. Moreover, the pallor of asphyxia pallida is corrected by oxygen therapy and assistance of ventilation, whereas the pallor associated with blood loss is improved only by correction of the anemia.

Treatment. Salvage of the infant who has sustained a major hemorrhage just prior to birth demands prompt recognition and correction of the deficit in blood volume. The opportunity to effect a cure may be lost by delay. Placement of an umbilical venous catheter permits monitoring of the central venous pressure and facilitates collection of blood for determinations of hemoglobin concentration and for blood typing and cross-match.

The infant's immediate need is expansion of the blood volume. This is best accomplished with whole blood. If the urgency of the situation obviates the delay inherent in obtaining properly cross-matched blood, the infant should be given blood drawn by syringe from a member of the immediately available delivery team who is known to have group-O, Rh (D)-negative blood. Clotting of blood collected in this fashion is prevented by moistening the barrel of the syringe with heparin. The administration of 20 ml. of whole blood per kilogram of body weight by rapid infusion is followed by immediate improvement of color and respiratory effort. Repeat transfusions of 10 ml./kg. may be given until the peripheral circulation is improved and a measurable central venous pressure is observed.

The infant with chronic or remote hemorrhage is generally well compensated. Because volume overload is a potential risk, blood should not be given.

Congestive heart failure secondary to severe anemia is best managed with a small exchange transfusion. The use of sedimented red cells instead of whole blood facilitates rapid correction of anemia and permits the creation of a volume deficit.

All infants with perinatal blood loss are particularly vulnerable to iron deficiency. It is recommended that they be given ferrous sulfate orally during the first year of life (5 mg. of elemental iron per kg. per day).

Anemia after the First Day of Life

In addition to isosensitization and fetal hemorrhage, other mechanisms for the genesis of anemia assume significance after the immediate neonatal period. Because hypochromic, microcytic anemias and macrocytic anemias are rarely encountered in the young infant, the traditional morphologic approach to differential diagnosis is not likely to prove helpful. Differentiation of the normochromic, normocytic anemias is facilitated by an assessment of red cell kinetics. Reticulocytosis, normoblastosis, poikilocytosis and polychromatophilia are expressions of accelerated red cell production. Increased destruction is reflected by an increase in serum unconjugated bilirubin. In interpreting the significance of hyperbilirubinemia it is necessary to consider the limited capacity of the liver for bilirubin conjugation during the first week of life. A diagnosis of hemolytic disease may be made if there is evidence for both accelerated red cell production and destruction. Increased red cell production without increased destruction indicates posthemorrhagic anemia. Hypoplasia of the erythroid marrow is responsible for the anemia which fails to provoke an increase in red cell production.

Because of the frequency with which jaundice is associated with anemia in the neonatal period, an investigation of red cell turnover is indicated if (1) jaundice is detected in the first 24 hours; (2) the serum bilirubin exceeds 12 mg./100 ml. in term infants or 15 mg./100 ml. in premature infants; or (3) clinically detectable jaundice persists beyond the first week of life. Nonphysiologic hyperbilirubinemia is observed with bleeding into soft tissues and with hemolytic disease; both conditions are associated with evidence of accelerated erythropoiesis.

Blood loss anemia. Bleeding into the head and the retroperitoneal space is characteristically occult. The former is associated with respiratory distress; the latter gives rise to an abdominal mass. Hyperbilirubinemia due to the breakdown of extravasated blood may be sufficient to necessitate an exchange transfusion. The diagnosis of blood loss anemia rests on the demonstration of blood outside the vascular space.

Anemia with infection. Neonatal infections are commonly associated with anemia. Because it is rarely severe, the anemia is not a dominant feature of the infant's total illness. The syndromes resulting from fetal infections with cytomegalovirus, *Toxoplasma gondii,* rubella virus and *Treponema pallidum* are associated with varying degrees of hemolysis, erythroid hypoplasia and blood loss. Bacterial sepsis effectively suppresses erythropoiesis and, in addition, may trigger intravascular coagulation. The latter process is associated with red cell fragmentation and hemolysis.

Hereditary spherocytosis. At least 50% of infants with hereditary spherocytosis experience exaggerated hyperbilirubinemia in the first week of life. Exchange transfusion may be necessary to maintain the serum bilirubin within an acceptable range. Splenomegaly is not a feature of the disease in early life. Anemia, if present, is mild. The diagnosis is suggested by finding microspherocytes in the peripheral blood smear. Sphering of the red cell is a feature of many hemolytic states (including ABO incompatibility); therefore this morphologic observation must be followed up with a study of in vitro hemolysis and a survey of family members. Microspherocytes and evidence for hemolysis will be observed in one parent and may be detected in one or more siblings. Red cells from the infant and affected family members undergo exaggerated spontaneous hemolysis when incubated under sterile conditions (autohemolysis test). The hemolysis is partially corrected by both glucose and ATP. Because of the risk of overwhelming infection in young children whose spleens are removed, this procedure is postponed until the fourth birthday. Although generally not necessary, transfusions of packed red cells may be given for severe or symptomatic anemia until the spleen is extirpated.

Nonspherocytic hemolytic anemia. Congenital hemolytic disorders not associated with abnormal red cell morphology are classified as congenital nonspherocytic hemolytic anemias. These are a heterogeneous group of inherited disorders which have in common deficient red cell glycolysis.

The most commonly encountered disorder of glycolysis results from an inherited deficiency of glucose-6-phosphate dehydrogenase (G-6-PD). This enzyme is necessary for the generation of NADPH and reduced glutathione. The latter protects the hemoglobin molecule from oxidative injury. If exposed to oxidant drugs or toxins, the hemoglobin in cells deficient in G-6-PD undergoes rapid and irreversible oxidation. Hemoglobin denatured by oxidative injury forms intracellular precipitates known as Heinz bodies. By attaching themselves to red cell membranes, Heinz bodies compromise erythrocyte deformability. Because rigid red cells are not able to negotiate the reticular meshwork of the spleen, they are removed from the circulation.

Deficiency of red cell G-6-PD is encountered primarily in populations which have migrated from the northern Mediterranean countries, southeastern Asia and Africa. A full 12% of American Negro males and 2-3% of Negro females are deficient in the enzyme. Although severe neonatal jaundice is observed in Caucasian and Mongoloid (Oriental) infants with G-6-PD deficiency, affected Negroes manifest no jaundice unless they are exposed to drugs or toxins with oxidant properties. The extensive list of offending agents includes sulfonamides, nitrofurantoin (Furadantin), salicylates, acetanilid, water-soluble vitamin K analogues (Synkavite, Hykinone), chloramphenicol, and naphthalene. Little or no anemia is observed unless an offending drug or toxin is implicated.

Heinz bodies are readily identified in supravitally stained preparations. The diagnosis is established by assay of enzyme activity in red cells. A G-6-PD "spot test" is useful for screening purposes; however, because the most deficient cells are preferentially removed from the circulation, a normal "spot test" after a hemolytic crisis does not exclude the diagnosis. The test should be repeated 1 to 2 months after recovery from the episode of hyperbilirubinemia.

Because of predominant Hb F synthesis in the neonatal period, those disorders which result from abnormalities of beta-chain synthesis do not express themselves until later. Thus, infants with beta-chain hemoglobinopathies (Hb S disease, Hb C disease) and infants destined to have beta-thalassemia (Cooley's anemia) are clinically and hematologically normal during the first 4 to 6 months of life.

COAGULATION DISORDERS

The diagnostic and therapeutic skill of the physician is not infrequently challenged by the infant with diffuse bleeding. Because of its immediate life-threatening implications, the hemostatic defect or defects must be promptly characterized and corrected. Orderliness in the plan of evaluation, economy in the use of blood for diagnostic purposes, and judicial interpretation of historical, clinical, and laboratory data are the essential prerequisites for effective management.

Before embarking on a diagnostic evaluation, the physician needs to be secure in his diagnosis of pathologic bleeding. The passage by rectum or mouth of swallowed maternal blood is often mistaken for fetal hemorrhage. The maternal origin of the blood is readily documented at the bedside by the Apt test. The bloody vomitus or meconium is mixed with 5 parts

of water in a test tube. After removal of particulate matter by centrifugation, 1 ml. of 0.25 N sodium hydroxide is added to 5 ml. of the pink
supernatant. Blood of maternal origin turns brown within 2 minutes,
whereas blood which contains predominantly Hb F remains pink.

Spontaneous bleeding in the newborn infant most commonly results
from one of three mechanisms: (1) vitamin K deficiency (hemorrhagic
disease of the newborn); (2) isolated thrombocytopenia; or (3) disseminated intravascular coagulation. Pathologic bleeding following surgery or
injury is seen in infants with congenital deficiencies of plasma coagulation factors.

Proper interpretation of coagulation studies requires conversance
with the physiologic alterations which characterize hemostasis in normal
infants. Cord blood is deficient in those plasma factors which are dependent on vitamin K: factors II (prothrombin), VII, IX and X. As a
result, both the partial thromboplastin time (PTT) and the prothrombin
time (PT) are prolonged relative to the standards established for older
subjects (Table 7-3). Although fibrinogen concentration is normal, the
thrombin time (TT) is also prolonged. The mechanism responsible for this
"heparin-like" activity of neonatal blood is unknown. Unless vitamin K
is given at birth, the increase in PTT and PT is progressive during the
first 2-4 days of life. The platelet count and levels of factors VIII, XII
and XIII are usually comparable to those found in normal adult plasma.
Factors V and XI, though often low in the neonatal period, are not responsible for clinically apparent defects of hemostasis.

Hemorrhagic Disease of the Newborn

Hemorrhagic disease of the newborn (HDNB) is a syndrome of
diffuse bleeding caused by deficiency of vitamin K and characterized by
low levels of factors II, VII, IX and X. Lacking stores of vitamin K and
the enteric flora necessary for vitamin K synthesis, the newborn infant
is dependent entirely on dietary supply of the vitamin to meet aug-
mented needs. Cow's milk contains enough vitamin K to meet the requirements of the neonate, but the vitamin K content of human milk
is often inadequate. As a result, breast-fed infants and infants unable to
tolerate oral feeding experience a progressive decrease in the coagulation

Table 7-3. COAGULATION STUDIES IN NEONATAL HEMORRHAGIC DISORDERS

Condition	PTT (sec.)	PT (sec.)	TT (sec.)	Fibrinogen (mg.)	Platelets (per mm.³)	FSP
Normal adult	37-50*	12-14	7-10	200-350	200,000-450,000	0
Normal neonate	44-80	12-20	8-20	120-250	150,000-400,000	±
HDNB	↑	↑	N	N	N	0
TCP	N	N	N	N	↓	0
DIC	↑↑	↑(N)	↑(N)	↓(N)	↓↓	+
Hemophilia	↑	N	N	N	N	0

PTT = activated partial thromboplastin time; PT = prothrombin time; TT = thrombin time; FSP = fibrin split products;
HDNB = hemorrhagic disease of the newborn; TCP = thrombocytopenia; DIC = disseminated intravascular coagulation;
N = normal. Arrows = above or below normal ranges.
*Values represent normal ranges.

factors that are dependent on vitamin K. By the second to fourth day of life the deficiency may be sufficient to permit spontaneous hemorrhage.

Neonatal vitamin K deficiency is characterized clinically by profuse bleeding from the gastrointestinal tract, umbilical cord, nose and sites of skin puncture. Typically, bleeding is first observed on the second or third day of life; rarely, the onset of bleeding is as early as the first day or as late as the fifth day of life. Hyperbilirubinemia, due to the absorption of heme pigments from sites of soft-tissue hemorrhage, may assume prominence after correction of the hemostatic defect.

The diagnosis of HDNB is based on (1) demonstration of a greatly prolonged PT and (2) correction of the PT by vitamin K. Although not so long as the PT, the PTT is also increased. The TT is within the normal neonatal range. Within 2 hours of vitamin K administration, bleeding stops. A decrease in the PT is observed by 4 hours. Twenty-four hours after treatment the PT should be within a normal range.

HDNB in the term infant is effectively treated by the intravenous injection of 1-2 mg. of vitamin K_1 (AquaMephyton, Konakion). Correction of vitamin K deficiency facilitates immediate hepatic synthesis of factors II, VII, IX and X. Infants whose liver function is compromised by immaturity or disease have a less predictable response to vitamin K. These infants are best treated with fresh-frozen plasma (10 ml. per kg.). Vitamin K should be given concomitantly.

HDNB is better prevented than treated. There is no contraindication to the prophylactic administration of 1 mg. of vitamin K_1 oxide at birth. Failure to incorporate this simple precaution into the routine care of newborn infants is attended by significant risk of hemorrhage. Sutherland observed a 5% risk of spontaneous bleeding in breast-fed infants not given vitamin K at birth. With circumcision the risk increased to 10%.

Thrombocytopenic Purpura

The hallmarks of thrombocytopenia (TCP) in the neonate, as in the older child, are petechiae and ecchymoses. Less frequently, deep hematomas are observed. The generalized, often elevated petechiae of TCP should not be confused with the innocent "stress" petechiae which are seen over the shoulders and face of nonthrombocytopenic infants. The latter lesions result from a temporary increase in superior vena caval pressure during vertex deliveries. Platelet counts less than 150,000/mm.^{3} should be considered abnormal in premature as well as in mature infants. The diagnostic possibilities suggested by isolated TCP are different from those invoked to explain TCP associated with other hemostatic defects. This section deals with those disorders characterized by isolated TCP.

Isoimmune neonatal thrombocytopenia. In a manner analogous to hemolytic disease due to fetal-maternal red cell incompatibility, neonatal TCP may result from fetal-maternal platelet incompatibility. Unlike isosensitization due to Rh (D) incompatibility, isoimmune TCP is not infrequently observed in the offspring of first pregnancies. Purpura, which is evident at birth, persists until the second to fourth month of life, when the transplacentally acquired antibody is exhausted. Intracranial bleeding, though rare, is a reported complication. The liver and spleen are normal in size. Bone marrow megakaryocytes are normal or increased in number.

The diagnosis of isoimmune neonatal TCP is documented by the demonstration of fetal-maternal platelet incompatibility and anti-platelet antibody in the affected infant. Unfortunately, reliable technics for platelet typing and platelet antibody detection are not generally available. A presumptive diagnosis can be made in an otherwise healthy thrombocytopenic infant whose mother has a normal platelet count. The diagnosis is strengthened if platelets from the mother survive normally in the infant. Platelets harvested from one unit of blood can be expected to increase the platelet count of the mature infant by 50,000/mm.^{3}. The half-life of transfused platelets is approximately 3 days.

Symptomatic isoimmune TCP is promptly corrected by maternal platelets (Adner et al.). Platelets harvested from random donors are not effective. There is no convincing evidence that corticosteroids decrease the risk of bleeding or speed the advent of remission.

Autoimmune neonatal thrombocytopenia. Idiopathic thrombocytopenic purpura (ITP) in the adult population usually results from platelet sensitization by an autoantibody. Because sensitized platelets are removed from the circulation by the spleen, splenectomy is often curative despite continued coating of platelets by antibody. The platelet antibody elaborated by women with ITP penetrates the placenta and coats fetal platelets. As a result, transient TCP is a predictable disorder of infants born to women with ITP or TCP secondary to lupus erythematosus. Infant platelets are innocent victims of the maternal autoimmune disorder. Generalized purpura is apparent at birth or shortly thereafter and persists until the maternal antibody is cleared from the infant's circulation (1-3 months). As with other neonatal hemorrhagic syndromes, hyperbilirubinemia may complicate soft-tissue bleeding during the first week of life. No associated defects are detected by clinical or laboratory evaluation. Marrow megakaryocytes are characteristically increased.

The diagnosis of autoimmune TCP may be made in the thrombocytopenic infant born to a mother with ITP. The maternal platelet count is decreased unless prior splenectomy has effected a hematologic remission. Neither splenectomy nor corticosteroids given to the mother protect the fetus.

The treatment of autoimmune neonatal TCP is difficult to evaluate. The vast majority of affected infants experience no significant bleeding, irrespective of the therapeutic program employed. Transfused platelets, whether from the mother or a random donor, are rapidly sensitized and are sequestered by the infant's spleen. Attempts to remove significant amounts of antibody by exchange transfusion have been unsuccessful. Although corticosteroids are commonly used, it is doubtful that they significantly alter the natural course of the disorder. The infant is best managed by careful, frequent examination. Should life-threatening hemorrhage occur, immediate splenectomy is indicated.

Thrombocytopenia with neonatal infections. TCP is a frequent complication of the survivors of fetal infection. Congenital cytomegalic inclusion disease, toxoplasmosis, rubella, syphilis and herpes simplex characteristically provoke thrombocytopenic purpura. The reported decrease of megakaryocytes in the marrows of infants with cytomegaloviral infections and the rubella syndrome suggests that decreased thrombopoiesis is responsible for at least some infection-associated TCP. Although it is a frequent feature of prenatally acquired infection, TCP rarely gives rise to significant bleeding. The significance of TCP in an infant with multisystemic disease lies not in its therapeutic implications but in its potential to facilitate recognition of the primary disorder.

Infrequent causes of neonatal thrombocytopenia. Knowledge of drug exposure is essential in the evaluation of TCP, regardless of the patient's age. Although drugs to which the neonate is exposed rarely produce TCP, drugs given to the mother may adversely affect the level of fetal platelets. Quinine, quinidine, Sedormid and sulfonamides may bind with platelets in such a fashion as to provoke the production of antibodies against the drug-platelet complex. These drugs cross the placental barrier; therefore fetal and maternal platelets are destroyed. Alternatively, drugs given the mother may suppress fetal thrombopoiesis. Although chlorthiazides have been incriminated as selective suppressants of fetal thrombopoiesis, recent surveys (Merenstein et al.) have failed to confirm the initial reports.

Congenital absence or decrease in bone marrow megakaryocytes is associated with skeletal anomalies, notably congenital absence of the radii. Thrombocytopenic purpura is a prominent feature of congenital leukemia, a diagnosis which is readily apparent from examination of the peripheral blood smear.

Disseminated Intravascular Coagulation

In recent years disseminated intravascular coagulation (DIC) has been recognized with increasing frequency as a cause of life-threatening hemorrhage in the neonatal period (Abildgaard; Hathaway et al., 1969). Evidence for disseminated fibrin thromboembolism is found in approximately 15% of infants dying between 2 and 28 days of age (Boyd). Activation of the clotting mechanism within the intact circulation is attended by three pernicious consequences: (1) depletion of those clotting factors which are consumed in the clotting process (platelets, fibrinogen, factors V and VIII); (2) widespread tissue necrosis due to the formation of thrombi in the microcirculation; and (3) fragmentation of red cell membranes by intravascular fibrin deposits. In response to fibrin deposition, physiologic mechanisms for fibrinolysis are activated. Fibrinolytic split products, in turn, potentiate the coagulopathy by interfering with the conversion of thrombin to fibrin.

DIC may be triggered by endotoxemia, by endothelial damage, by the escape of tissue thromboplastin into the circulation or by platelet aggregation. More often, however, the mechanism responsible for activation of the clotting cascade is not apparent. Almost always, the infant is stressed by an underlying disease. DIC may complicate a host of congenital and neonatally acquired infections, respiratory distress syndrome, cyanotic congenital heart disease, cavernous hemangiomas, amniotic fluid embolization, intrauterine asphyxia, maternal toxemia, abruptio placentae, postmaturity, shock and severe acidosis.

The most impressive clinical expression of DIC is pathologic bleeding. Rapid consumption of platelets and clotting factors (acute DIC) is associated with widespread hemorrhages in the skin, mucous membranes and viscera. Not infrequently death results from intracranial bleeding. With more dilatory consumption (chronic DIC), the synthetic rates for factors II, V and VIII and for platelets are not exceeded. Although tests of hemostasis are abnormal, spontaneous bleeding is not observed. The microthrombi associated with both acute and chronic DIC are responsible for varying degrees of tissue necrosis and hemolysis. Consequently, functional impairment of the liver, kidneys or brain is commonly observed. Anemia, with or without jaundice, results in part from blood loss and in part from mechanical disruption of red cells by meshes of intravascular fibrin.

There is no unanimity of opinion regarding the essential diagnostic criteria for DIC. Several of the tests which are helpful in demonstrating DIC in older subjects are of little or no value in the neonate. For example, fibrin split products are detected by sensitive technics in approximately 60% of normal neonates during the first 24 hours of life (Stiehm et al.). These degradation products are probably derived from the lysis of placental clots. Moreover, the PT and TT, both of which are abnormal in DIC, are prolonged in the normal neonate. Until more sensitive and reliable diagnostic methods are developed, it is recommended that three essential criteria be met before a diagnosis of DIC is made: (1) severe thrombocytopenia or a rapidly falling platelet count; (2) morphologic evidence for red cell fragmentation—that is, the demonstration of burr cells, helmet cells, spherocytes and fragments of red cells (schistocytes) in the peripheral blood smear; and (3) prolonged PT. After the first day of life, detection of fibrinolytic split products assumes significance. The most sensitive technics for detection of split products are the hemagglutination-inhibition of fibrinogen-coated, tanned red cells and the staphylococcal clumping tests. Euglobulin lysis and protamine sulfate precipitation tests are too insensitive to have much clinical utility. The PTT and TT are usually, though not necessarily, prolonged. Levels of factors V and VIII are decreased. The fibrinogen concentration is typically decreased but may be normal.

Heparin is the mainstay of therapy for DIC in older children and adults (Hathaway, 1970). This anticoagulant effectively arrests intravascular clotting and thereby facilitates restoration of those factors which are consumed by the clotting process. Unfortunately, the administration of heparin to the neonate is attended by significant obstacles. The metabolic fate of heparin in the newborn infant is uncertain, the dose necessary to achieve therapeutic heparinization is highly variable, and the technics necessary for monitoring heparin effect are not readily applied to the small infant. Moreover, once the consumption is arrested by heparin the neonate does not regenerate coagulation factors with the efficiency of older subjects; as a result, the therapeutic effect of heparin is less predictable. Finally, there is no convincing evidence at present that heparin improves the survival of newborn infants with DIC. On the other hand, the risk of magnifying hemorrhage by over-use of heparin is real.

It is not possible to define a set of therapeutic recommendations which can be applied to all infants with DIC. However, certain guiding principles emerge:

1. Treat the underlying disease which is responsible for DIC. Correction of shock, acidosis and hypoxia may remove the triggering mechanism for DIC. The survival of infants with DIC secondary to bacteremia is a function of the success with which the infection, not the coagulopathy, is treated.

2. Treat the patient, not the abnormal laboratory tests. Chronic DIC, unassociated with clinical bleeding or complications of microangiopathy, is best managed with diligent observation and restraint.

3. Avoid replacing platelets and coagulation factors unless consumption has been arrested. Platelets, fibrinogen and factor VIII given to the patient with consumptive coagulopathy do little more than add fuel to the fire. Such therapy extends thrombosis in the microcirculation without improving hemostasis.

4. Perform an exchange transfusion if the infant with documented DIC experiences spontaneous bleeding. This procedure temporarily arrests consumption and replaces those factors which are exhausted. It is imperative that fresh whole blood be used. Although heparinized donor blood is to be preferred, citrated blood has been used with favorable results (Gross et. al.).

5. Do not give the infant heparin unless exchange transfusion has proved unsuccessful and unless the facilities and personnel necessary

for diligent monitoring of heparin effect are available. Intravenous administration of heparin is best done by means of a constant-infusion pump. During the first 4 hours, 100 units of heparin per kilogram of body weight are infused. The rate of administration thereafter is determined by the results of clotting studies. The activated PTT should be maintained at 80-100 seconds or the clotting time at 20-40 minutes. Once the full effect of heparin has been achieved, some infants require no more than 10-20 units of heparin per day in order to maintain a full therapeutic effect. Other infants require much larger amounts. Heparin is continued until the underlying disease process is corrected.

Hemophilia

Deficiencies of factors VIII and IX account for 90% of the congenital disorders of blood coagulation. Both disorders are transmitted as X-linked recessive traits, and both predispose to pathologic bleeding in muscles, joints and other deep structures. Spontaneous bleeding in mucous membranes and excessive bleeding from superficial cuts and abrasions are not observed. Because infants are infequently subjected to injury, the defect is often not apparent until after the neonatal period. On the other hand, abnormal bleeding after circumcision may be the first indication of the hemostatic defect. At least a third of hemophiliacs do not experience excessive bleeding with circumcision.

The diagnosis of a first-stage clotting defect is based on a prolonged PTT associated with a normal PT. The clotting time is not recommended as a screening test for hemophilia. Because concentrates used in the treatment of factor-VIII deficiency contain no factor IX and because factor-IX concentrates contain no factor VIII, it is essential that the first-stage clotting defect be further characterized. A presumptive diagnosis of factor-VIII deficiency is made if plasma known to be deficient in factor IX corrects the abnormal PTT. Correction of the PTT by plasma deficient in factor VIII suggests factor-IX deficiency. The diagnosis is confirmed by assay of factor-VIII or factor-IX activity.

Control of bleeding necessitates replacement of the deficient factor. Effective hemostasis is achieved with a factor-VIII or factor-IX level of 30% (normal 50-200%). For most soft-tissue bleeding this level is maintained for 48 hours. Maintenance of good hemostatic levels for longer periods is necessary in intracranial hemorrhage and other life-threatening bleeding episodes. One unit of factor VIII (that amount contained in 1 ml. of plasma) per kilogram of body weight increases factor-VIII activity by approximately 2%. One unit of factor IX/kg. increases factor-IX activity by 1%. The half-life of transfused factor VIII is approximately 10 hours, that of factor IX approximately 30 hours. With this information one can calculate the amount of factor VIII or factor IX which need be given. Soft-tissue bleeding due to factor-VIII deficiency is readily arrested by the intravenous infusion of the contents of a single vial (250 units) of a factor-VIII concentrate. Minor bleeding resulting from factor-IX deficiency is satisfactorily treated with a single injection of 200 units of factor IX (Konyne) or with fresh-frozen plasma (5 ml. per pound of body weight every 12 hours for 24-36 hours). For a more detailed discussion of the management of the infant with hemophilia, the reader is referred to the useful handbook prepared by Strauss.

SUGGESTED READINGS

1. Abildgaard, C. F.: Recognition and treatment of intravascular coagulation, J. Pediat. 74:163, 1969.
2. Adner, M. M., et al.: Use of "compatible" platelet transfusions in treatment of congenital isoimmune thrombocytopenic purpura, New England J. Med. 280:244, 1969.
3. Allen, F. H., and Diamond, L. K.: *Erythroblastosis Fetalis* (Boston: Little, Brown & Co., 1957).
4. Bowman, J. M., et al.: Fetal transfusion in severe Rh isoimmunization. Indications, efficiency, and results based on 218 transfusions carried out on 100 fetuses, J.A.M.A. 207:1101, 1969.
5. Bowman, J. M., and Friesen, R. F.: Hemolytic Disease of the Newborn, in Gellis, S. S., and Kagan, B. M. (ed.): *Current Pediatric Therapy* (4th ed.; Philadelphia: W. B. Saunders Company, 1970).
6. Boyd, J. F.: Disseminated fibrin thromboembolism among neonates dying more than 48 hours after birth, J. Clin. Path. 22:663, 1969.
7. Cohen, F., et al.: Mechanisms of isoimmunication. I. The transplacental passage of fetal erythrocytes in homospecific pregnancies, Blood 23:621, 1964.
8. Fogel, B. J., Arias, D., and Kung, F: Platelet counts in healthy premature infants, J. Pediat. 73:108, 1968.

9. Gross, S., and Melhorn, D. K.: Exchange transfusion with citrated whole blood for disseminated intravascular coagulation, J. Pediat. 78:415, 1971.

10. Guest, G. M., and Brown, E. W.: Erythrocyte and hemoglobin of the blood in infancy and childhood. III. Factors in variability, statistical studies, Am. J. Dis. Child. 93:486, 1957.

11. Hathaway, W. E., Mull, M. M., and Pechet, G. S.: Disseminated intravascular coagulation in the newborn, Pediatrics 43:233, 1969.

12. Hathaway, W. E.: Care of the critically ill child: The problem of disseminated intravascular coagulation, Pediatrics 46:767, 1970.

13. Kirkman, H. N., and Riley, H. D.: Posthemorrhagic anemia and shock in the newborn: A review, Pediatrics 24:97, 1959.

14. Mauer, A. M.: *Pediatric Hematology* (New York: McGraw-Hill Book Co., 1969).

15. Medoff, H. S.: Platelet counts in premature infants, J. Pediat. 64: 287, 1964.

16. Merenstein, G. B., O'Loughlin, E. P., and Plunket, D. C.: Effects of maternal thiazides on platelet counts of newborn infants, J. Pediat. 76:766, 1970.

17. Odell, G. B., Cohen, S. N., and Gordes, E. H.: Administration of albumin in the management of hyperbilirubinemia by exchange transfusions, Pediatrics 30:613, 1962.

18. Oski, F. A., and Naiman, J. L.: *Hematologic Problems in the Newborn* (2d ed.; Philadelphia: W. B. Saunders Company, 1972).

19. Oski, F. A., et al: The effects of deoxygenation of adult and fetal hemoglobin on the synthesis of red cell 2,3-diphosphoglycerate and its in vivo consequences, J. Clin. Invest. 49:400, 1970.

20. Pochedly, C.: The exchange transfusion: Newer concepts and advances in technic, Clin. Pediat. 7:383, 1968.

21. Pollack, W., et al.: Results of clinical trials of RhoGAM in women, Transfusions 8:151, 1968.

22. Raye, J. R., Gutberlet, R. L., and Stahlman, M.: Symptomatic posthemorrhagic anemia in the newborn, Pediat. Clin. North America 17:401, 1970.

23. Stiehm, E. R., and Clatanoff, D. V.: Split products of fibrin in the serum of newborns, Pediatrics 43:770, 1969.

24. Strauss, H. S:: *Diagnosis and Treatment of Hemophilia. A Practical Guide* (3d ed.; Albany: Albany Medical College, 1972).

25. Sutherland, J. M., Glueck, H. I., and Gleser, G.: Hemorrhagic disease of the newborn. Breast feeding as a necessary factor in the pathogenesis, Am. J. Dis. Child. 113:524, 1967.

CHAPTER 8

Infections of the Newborn Infant

G. VAN LEEUWEN, M.D.

The incidence of generalized infection of the newborn is extremely difficult to establish. In hospitals where the obstetric population is not at risk the total incidence may be as low as 2 per 1,000 deliveries. In nurseries where high-risk pregnancies are commonly encountered the incidence may be as high as 12-15 per 1,000 deliveries.

GENERAL CONSIDERATIONS

Infection of the newborn is most easily understood if it is divided into three categories: prenatal, intranatal and postnatal.

1. Prenatal infection implies that the organism which has affected the fetus has come from the mother and has crossed the placental barrier. The most striking examples of this type of septicemia, at present, are cytomegaloviral and rubella infections.

2. Intranatal infection occurs secondary to rupture of the amniotic membranes. The affected infants become ill in the first 24 hours of life; often they are ill from the moment of birth. The organisms encountered in this type of infection are varied; gram-positive and gram-negative organisms are present with almost equal frequency.

3. Postnatally acquired septicemia is that which becomes evident in the infant beyond 24 hours of life and is usually the result of exposure to organisms acquired from other infants, from hospital personnel or from nursery equipment. The incidence of postnatal septicemia is closely related to technics and policies in any given nursery unit.

In this chapter the three forms of septicemia will be briefly described with respect to significance and recognition; then treatment and outcome will be described; and, lastly, immunoglobulin levels and their value will be discussed briefly.

It was originally hoped that measuring cord blood IGM levels, or later levels, might be useful in the detection of infants infected in utero. Unfortunately, there are too many false negatives to make the test reliable for screening. False negatives result from delayed antibody response and the short duration of elevation in some infants.

We use IGM levels in a select group of infants: those who are of low birthweight for their gestational age, those who do not thrive appropriately in the neonatal period, those who have detectable abnormal neurologic behavior, and those with unexplained petechiae or purpura, ocular findings and hepatosplenomegaly. In this way we have diagnosed a number of infants with cytomegaloviral and rubella infections who might otherwise have been undetected.

Prenatal Infection

Although all infections in the mother during pregnancy have a potentially adverse effect on the newborn infant, much more is known about some infections than others. With certain rare exceptions, the classic example of which is congenital syphilis, most neonatal involvement is secondary to viral infections in the mother. We now know, because of experience with the rubella virus, that the critical period for infection is the eighth to twelfth weeks of pregnancy.

By far the most common virus to affect the neonate is one of the herpes viruses, the cytomegalovirus. Next most common is the rubella virus. Other viral infections affecting the newborn are, as far as is known today, rare. Viral agents and the diseases they produce are listed in Table 8-1.

Cytomegalovirus and congenital rubella have in common a number of signs and symptoms in the newborn infant. These include low birthweight, hepatomegaly, splenomegaly, petechiae and purpura (Fig 8-1). Jaundice is more common in cytomegalic inclusion disease; congenital heart disease and cataracts are more common in rubella. Unfortunately, no treatment is effective for either of these diseases. The estimated incidence of cytomegaloviral disease is 6-15 per 1,000 live births; of rubella, 1-7 per 1,000. Of significance is the need to isolate from hospital personnel all infants who have evidence of rubella infection.

Table 8-1. VIRAL AGENTS OF FETAL AND NEONATAL DISEASE*

Agent	Disease
Myxoparamyxovirus	Abortion
Influenza	Psychomotor retardation
Mumps	? Endocardial fibroelastosis
	Abortion
Measles	Congenital measles
Herpesvirus	Subclinical-mild-severe congenital infections
Cytomegalovirus	Microcephaly, chorioretinitis, deafness, psychomotor disorders, mental retardation
Herpevirus hominis (simplex)	Disseminated neonatal infections
	? Congenital malformations (microcephaly, retinal dysplasia
Varicella-zoster (chickenpox-shingles)	Abortion
	Congenital varicella-zoster
Poxvirus	Abortion
Variola (smallpox)	Congenital smallpox
	Abortion
Vaccinia	Congenital generalized vaccinia
Picornavirus	Abortion
Poliovirus	Congenital poliomyelitis
	Subclinical neonatal infections, diarrhea
ECHO	Subclinical-mild-severe neonatal infections
Coxsackie	? Congenital heart disease, myocarditis
Arbovirus	Congenital encephalomyelitis
Western equine encephalomyelitis	
Eastern equine encephalomyelitis	
Other	Abortion
Rubella	Subclinical-mild-severe congenital infections
	Congenital malformations (congenital heart disease, cataracts, microcephaly, deafness, psychomotor retardation
Hepatitis (serum)	Neonatal hepatitis

*From Overall, J. C., and Glasgow, L. A.: Virus infections of the fetus and newborn infant, J. Pediat. 77:315, 1970.

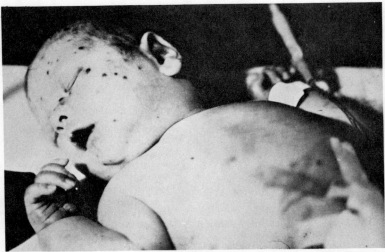

Fig. 8-1.—Infant with acute cytomegaloviral disease. Note moribund appearance, petechiae and purpura. Hepatosplenomegaly and anemia were also present. The baby expired at age 4 hours.

Congenital toxoplasmosis is also difficult to differentiate from cytomegalic inclusion disease. There is, however, a much higher incidence of retinopathy and cerebral calcifications in toxoplasmosis.

Infants who become infected with Coxsackie B virus often have severe disseminated disease involving multiple organs. Early in the neonatal period the disease has been known to run a particularly fulminating course, often resulting in death. Hyperthermia, hypothermia, lethargy, anorexia, vomiting, respiratory distress, cyanosis, cardiac disease and hepatosplenomegaly are all very common in the Coxsackie B infections, as well as in herpes simplex infections. There is evidence that there may also be a mild or asymptomatic form of Coxsackie B infection. We have seen a small group of infants in whom the primary sign of illness was a mild carditis and who recovered in 4 or 5 days.

Serious illness in the newborn secondary to herpes simplex infection has been much more recently described. In most cases infection seems to occur during passage through the vagina. The infant becomes ill during the first week of life. As with the Coxsackie B virus, many systems are involved; hence most of these infants are initally treated as having bacterial sepsis. The appearance of vesicles in clusters is helpful for the diagnosis.

The diagnosis of this type of septicemia is best established by isolating the virus from the infected infant. Serologic studies also offer some assistance. IGG readily crosses the placenta; therefore a titer in the infant will be the same as the titer in the mother. An elevated IGM level is significant; however, the test has many pitfalls (discussed below).

The therapy of viral infections in the newborn has been very discouraging. Idoxuridine and interferon have not become available commercially or are still investigational. The physician is left with the use of gamma globulin as the only effective chemotherapeutic agent against neonatal viral infections. Unfortunately, in most neonatal infections the disease is beyond the viremic phase before clinical illness becomes apparent, and therefore the use of gamma globulin is of very little value.

We have treated one newborn with disseminated herpes simplex infection with cyostine arabinoside, with eventual recovery (normal at 1 yr.).

Intranatal Infection

As previously mentioned, intranatal infection is usually acquired by ascending infection secondary to rupture of the amniotic membranes. Most of organisms in this instance are gram-negative bacteria, but gram-positive bacteria (chiefly enterococcal) are also found. The length of time the membranes have been ruptured and the amount of therapy which has been given to the mother are of little consequence to the infected neonate. So many exceptions occur, however, that for any given situation it is best to ignore both the duration of rupture and the extent of therapy.

Infected amniotic fluid may be suggested prior to delivery if the mother becomes febrile for no other explainable reason, if the fetus has a tachycardia in excess of 180/minute or if the amniotic fluid becomes meconium-stained, indicating distress in the neonate.

At the time of birth, evidence of infection is usually readily obtained. The physician should be suspicious if the infant is meconium-

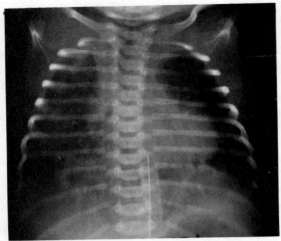

Fig. 8-2.—Pneumonia of the right lung, due to infected amniotic fluid. This is an example of intranatally acquired infection.

stained or if he smells bad at the time of birth. Because the respiratory cilia are active in utero, respiratory distress is the most frequent finding in intranatal sepsis (Fig. 8-2).

Other methods have been used to confirm the presence of infection at birth; these have included the examination of a frozen section of the umbilical cord. By and large these studies are time-consuming and not informative. The presence of polymorphonuclear leukocytes in the gastric aspirate at birth is said to be a meaningful indicator of which infants may become septic. We have found that if the number of white cells in an uncentrifuged specimen exceeds 5 per high-power field, the infant probably is infected. Culturing is done on all of these infants, and the infant with polymorphonuclear leukocytes in the gastric aspirate is observed with extreme care; however, he is not treated with antibiotics. The presence of organisms in the gastric aspirate is sufficiently common to be insignificant and of no clinical value.

The therapy of intranatal septicemia is identical with that of postnatal septicemia and will be discussed later.

Postnatal Septicemia

Postnatal septicemia usually becomes evident between 48 and 72 hours of life, although it may present earlier or later. The organisms supposedly are acquired from hospital personnel, from other infants or from the nursery equipment. Contrary to what was believed for many years, newborn infants do have signs and symptoms when they become infected, and therefore they should never receive prophylactic antibiotics. The most helpful clinical findings are respiratory distress, jaundice, anorexia and lethargy. A white blood count above 12,000 is frequently found. Any signs and symptoms may be present; the frequency of the most familiar of these is shown in Table 8-2. Distressing to all practitioners of newborn medicine is the fact that about 5-10% of infected infants are essentially asymptomatic.

Cellulitis of the umbilical area as an example of postnatal sepsis is shown in Figure 8-3. Figure 8-4 is an example of severe staphylococcal osteomyelitis following generalized septicemia in a 10-day-old infant.

Table 8-2. SIGNS AND SYMPTOMS MOST FREQUENTLY ASSOCIATED WITH SEPTICEMIA

Clinical Finding	Percentage of Infants
Respiratory distress Jaundice Elevated WBC (above 12,000) Refusal to feed	40-50
Lethargy Fever Hepatomegaly Apnea Cyanosis Vomiting	20-40
Hypothermia Abdominal distention Diarrhea Irritability	10-20
Asymptomatic	10

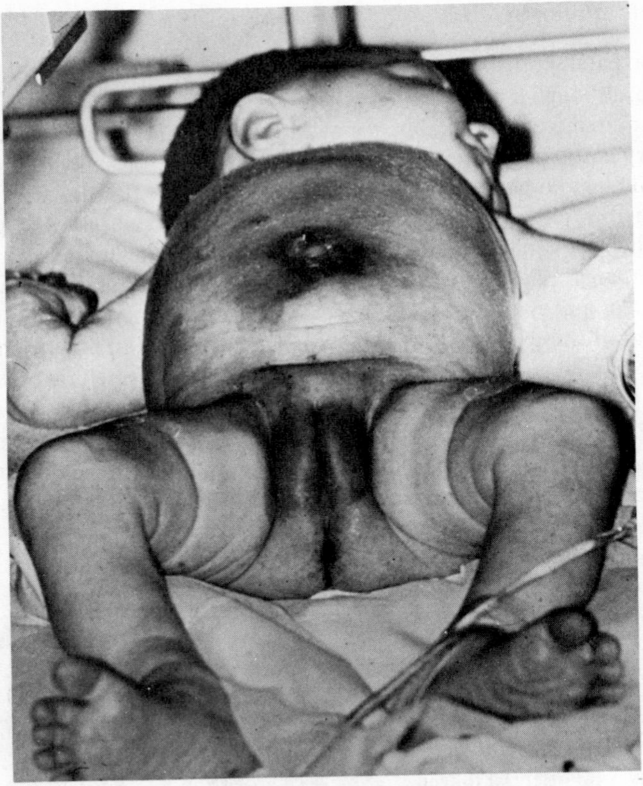

Fig. 8-3.–An unusual example of postnatal infection. The infant was delivered at home; the cord was cut with a razor blade and tied with string. The infant had severe abdominal cellulitis and streptococcal septicemia. The baby was hospitalized at age 9 days and died 24 hours later, in spite of vigorous therapy.

In newborn centers the diagnosis of septicemia is made clinically much more often than it is proven bacteriologically. A number of reasons for this have been proposed. Is it because of the likelihood that the infection was a viremia rather than bacteremia? Were improper culture technics or insufficient culturing sites used? Was the infant reacting to cold in the same way he reacts to infection? Infants with narcotic withdrawal symptoms and neurometabolic disease are commonly suspected of having septicemia and may die without appropriate diagnosis. We do not yet have answers to these questions. It is clear, however, that for every 10 infants in whom septicemia is clinically suspected, definitive bacteriologic proof is found in only approximately three.

Specific diagnostic procedures should be insisted upon whenever an infant is suspected of having bacterial septicemia. These include chest x-ray and cultures of the throat, anus, blood, cerebrospinal fluid and urine. When all of these areas are cultured the likelihood of recovering the offending organism is much improved. We have been impressed with the number of times the organism can only be identified in either the spinal fluid or the urine—and these happen to be the two areas most often ignored in the culturing procedures. To avoid needless delay, suprapubic aspiration for urine is now routine.

THERAPY AND OUTCOME

When an infant is suspected clinically of having septicemia and appropriate cultures have been taken, whether to institute therapy at once

Fig. 8-4.—Term infant who had generalized staphylococcal septicemia. He also developed osteomyelitis of the left proximal tibia, shown here.

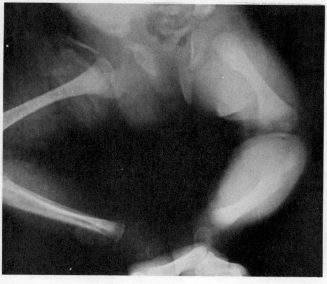

or to wait for culture results is a matter of clinical judgement. In our experience it is best to be rather vigorous in treating infants in whom one suspects sepsis. But one should remember that many antibiotics used in treating the newborn infant have had tragic results in the past; examples of this are chloromycetin and tetracyline. For years we used a combination of aqueous penicillin and kanamycin initially and thereafter converted to more appropriate antibiotics, depending upon the culture sensitivity. Recently, however, we have changed our format, for a number of reasons. We still recommend kanamycin 7-15 mg./kg./day, with the smaller dose for the small infant, given intramuscularly in 2-3 divided doses. As a second drug we use ampicillin, always intravenously during the acute stage of the illness and then intramuscularly every 6-8 hours. We presently use a 100-mg./kg. dosage. Ampicillin has replaced penicillin for a number of reasons, including its apparent safety in the newborn as well as a presumed synergistic effect with kanamycin.

It should be remembered that infants who are ill do not tolerate or absorb antibiotics orally. These drugs should always be given parenterally. When the infant has recovered fully but continuation of antibiotics is felt to be necessary for a time, conversion to oral medication may be made.

We may have to re-examine our concept of the treatment of sepsis in the light of the discovery of new antibiotics. Two seem particularly promising: colistin and gentamicin.

As indicated in the discussion, some neonatal viral infections are mild and some result in death. Especially dangerous are overwhelming cytomegaloviral and herpes simplex infections and many Coxsackie infections.

Even with prompt recognition of signs and symptoms and prompt institution of therapy, the mortality in bacterial septicemia approximates 25%. As one might expect, the death rate is higher in the infant at risk and highest in the infant who has undergone operative procedures.

SUGGESTED READINGS

1. Birnbaum, G., Lynch, J. I., Margileth, A. M., Lonergan, W. M., and Sever, J. L.: Cytomegalovirus infections in newborn infants, J. Pediat. 75:789, 1969.

2. Brown, G. C.: Recent advances in the viral aetiology of congenital anomalies, Advances Teratol. 1:55, 1966.
3. Buetow, K. C., Klein, S. W., and Lane, R. B.: Septicemia in premature infants, Am. J. Dis. Child. 110:29, 1965.
4. Burch, G. E., Sun, C. C., Chu, K. C., Sohal, R. S., and Colcolough, H. L.: Interstitial and Coxsackie B myocarditis in infants and children, J.A.M.A. 203:55, 1968.
5. Charnock, E. L., and Cramblett, H. G.: 5-iodo-2'-deoxyuridine in neonatal herpes virus hominis encephalitis, J. Pediat. 76:459, 1970.
6. Cherry, J. D., Soriano, F., and Jahn, C. L.: Search for perinatal viral infection: A prospective clinical virological and serological study, Am. J. Dis. Child. 116:245, 1968.
7. Eichenwald, H. F., and Shinefield, H. R.: Viral infections of the fetus and of the premature and newborn infant, Advances Pediat. 12:249, 1961.
8. Eichenwald, H. F., McCracken, G. H., Jr., and Kindberg, S. J.: Virus infections of the newborn, Progr. M. Virol. 9:35, 1967.
9. Feldman, R. A.: Cytomegalovirus infection during pregnancy, Am. J. Dis. Child. 117:517, 1969.
10. Gluck, L., Wood, H. F., and Fousek, M. D.: Septicemia in the newborn, Pediat. Clin. North America 13:1131, 1966.
11. Hall, C. B., and Miller, D. G.: The detection of a silent Coxsackie B-5 virus perinatal infection, J. Pediat. 75:124, 1969.
12. Hardy, J. B., McCracken, G. H., Gilkeson, M. R., and Sever, J. L.: Adverse fetal outcome following maternal rubella after the first trimester of pregnancy, J.A.M.A. 207:2414, 1969.
13. Hildebrandt, R. J., Sever, J. L., Margileth, A. M., and Callagan, D. A.: Cytomegalovirus in the normal pregnant woman, Am. J. Obst. & Gynec. 98:1125, 1967.
14. Horstmann, D. M.: Viral infections in pregnancy, Yale J. Biol. 42:99, 1969.
15. Isaacs, A., and Lindenman, J.: Virus interference. I. Interferon, Proc. Roy Soc. (Biol.) 147:258, 1957.
16. Jenning, R. C.: Coxsackie group B fatal neonatal myocarditis associated with cardiomegaly, Am. J. Clin. Path. 19:325, 1966.
17. McCracken, G. H., Jr., Hardy, J. B., Chen, T. C., Hoffman, L. S., Gilkeson, M. R., and Sever, J. L.: Serum immunoglobulin levels in newborn infants. II. Survey of cord and follow up sera from 123 infants with congenital rubella, J. Pediat. 74:383, 1969.
18. Moloshok, R. E.: Fetal risk associated with maternal systemic infections, Clin. Obst. & Gynec. 9:608, 1966.
19. Monif, G. R. G.: Viral Infections of the Human Fetus (London: Collier-Macmillan, Ltd., 1969).

20. Moorman, R. S., and Sell, S. A.: Neonatal septicemia, South. M. J. 54:137, 1961.
21. Nahmias, A. J., Josey, W. E., and Naib, Z. M.: Neonatal herpes simplex infection: Role of genital infection in mother as the source of virus in the newborn, J.A.M.A., 199:164, 1967.
22. Nahmias, A. J., Dowdle, W. R., Josey, W. E., Naib, Z. M., Painter, L. M., and Luce, C.: Newborn infection with herpesvirus hominis types 1 and 2, J. Pediat. 75:1194, 1969.
23. Nyhan, W. L., and Fousek, M. D.: Septicemia of the newborn, Pediatrics 22:268, 1958.
24. Overall, J. C., and Glasgow, L. A.: Virus infections of the fetus and newborn infant, J. Pediat. 77:315, 1970.
25. Sanders, D. Y., and Cramblett, H. G.: Viral infections in hospitalized neonates, Am. J. Dis. Child. 116:251, 1968.
26. Sever, J. L.: Immunological responses to perinatal infections, J. Pediat. 75:1116, 1292, 1969.
27. Sever, J. L., Hardy, J. B., Nelson, K. B., and Gilkeson, M. R.: Rubella in the collaborative perinatal research study, Am. J. Dis. Child. 118:123, 1969.
28. Sieber, O. F., Jr., Fulginiti, V. A., Brazie, J., and Umlauf, H. J., Jr.: In utero infection of the fetus by herpes simplex virus, J. Pediat. 69:30, 1966.
29. Silverman, W. A., and Homan, W. E.: Sepsis of obscure origin in the newborn, Pediatrics 3:157, 1949.
30. Smith, R. T., Platou, E. S., and Good, R. A.: Septicemia of the newborn; current status of the problem, Pediatrics 17:549, 1956.

CHAPTER 9

Hypoglycemia in the Newborn

R. A. GUTHRIE, M.D.

Carbohydrate is an important source of energy for a large number of cellular metabolic processes. In man the carbohydrate of greatest utility is glucose. Tissues vary greatly in their carbohydrate content—particularly in their use of glucose. This variation is due to the different energy requirements of organs and tissues and their ability to use other substrates, such as fatty acids.

The liver and the brain are prime examples of the need for glucose. The liver not only uses glucose in the metabolism of its cells but can make glucose from other substrates and can store it, as glycogen. The brain can neither make glucose nor store glycogen, nor can it metabolize other substrates except in very limited quantities and under very special circumstances. The brain is therefore dependent for its energy source on a constant supply of circulating glucose. Heart and muscle are intermediate: they can store glycogen and release it as glucose, and they can use other energy sources in limited amounts but cannot make glucose from other sources. The blood glucose level, then, is in dynamic equilibrium between glucose input from dietary intake, glucose release by liver and muscle, gluconeogenesis by liver and kidney and glucose uptake by the peripheral tissues—primarily brain, heart, muscle and adipose tissue. A complex set of enzymatic and hormonal interrelationships control these processes.

GLUCOSE ACQUISITION BY THE FETUS

Glucose is a major source of energy for the fetus. The fetus receives a constant supply of glucose from the mother via the placenta. The placenta must transfer 10-20 mg. of glucose per minute to the term fetus. Because glucose in the mother and fetus follows a concentration gradient, placental transfer of glucose is probably by diffusion. Placental transfer of glucose, however, is somewhat more complicated than simple diffusion. This is indicated by the fact that fructose, with the same molecular weight as glucose, does not cross the placenta as rapidly as does glucose. Facilitated diffusion of glucose has been suggested; i.e., there may be mechanisms to facilitate a faster rate of transfer of glucose than would be predicted on physiochemical grounds alone. Stereospecificity may play a role in facilitated diffusion. Levels of glucose in fetal blood do not exceed those of the mother; again, this suggests that transfer is not entirely by classical active-transport mechanisms. With facilitated diffusion, the cellular energy needed for growth and development—particularly the needs of the brain—would be protected even in the presence of maternal levels of glucose that would be below the optimum diffusion gradient levels. In the presence of placental malfunction, as in toxemia of pregnancy and other placental insufficiency states or anoxia of the placenta, there may be loss of this facilitated diffusion capability, and decreased glucose transfer from mother to fetus may result.

BLOOD GLUCOSE LEVELS IN NORMAL NEWBORNS

In order to assess the presence or effect of hypoglycemia in the neonate, one must first know what constitutes normal blood sugar levels. There is some disagreement in the literature as to what constitutes the upper and lower levels of normal for blood glucose; this is because a host of factors provide important variables, which have not been well standardized in many studies. The age of the infant, the sampling technic and frequency, the period of fasting, chilling of the infant and the method of determining blood glucose are some of these variables.

The proper handling of specimens for glucose analysis should include the immediate preparation of a protein-free filtrate by the Somogyi technic (see Suggested Readings) to stop red cell glycolysis. The sample should then be analyzed by Teller's glucose oxidase method for true glucose values.

An alternative method of glucose determination is the use of the Dextrostix and a reflectance meter. In our hands the Dextrostix alone has proven to be a reasonably reliable screening tool but has not been sufficiently reliable for definitive studies. Proper technics must be observed. This method offers the advantage of a quick blood glucose determination on

Table 9-1. BLOOD SUGAR LEVELS IN TERM NEONATES*

Authors	Cord	½	1	2	3	4	6	9	12	24	48	96
							Age (Hours)					
Creery and Parkinson	80	60	51	52	56		56	52	52			
Farquhar	76	77	71	64		63	63			66	65	73
Cornblath and Reesnor	66	55	55	48	52	55	47			57	57	69
Guthrie et al.	70	58	54				46	45	46	54	58	72
Norval										55	57	68

*From Cornblath, M., and Schwartz, R.: Disorders of Carbohydrate Metabolism (Philadelphia: W. B. Saunders Company, 1966), passim.

a capillary sample. Error with the Dextrostix usually occurs with over-washing or delayed reading, and both errors tend to give values lower than the true glucose values. The errors are in the right direction for protection of the infant's brain from hypoglycemia, but they do result in over-diagnosis and unnecessary treatment. When proper technics are used the Dextrostix-reflectance meter system has given correct blood glucose values within $\pm$ 5 mg./100 ml. when compared with glucose oxidase or autoanalyzer methods. Blood sugar levels should be confirmed in the laboratory.

Normal values for blood glucose in the neonate at various ages are shown in Table 9-1. Before feedings are initiated, in the first 6-12 hours of life, the blood glucose fluctuates widely; mean values are about 50-60 mg./100 ml. Once feedings have begun, mean blood glucose values tend to rise, even if the infant is deprived of food for several hours before the blood sample is obtained.

The definition of hypoglycemia in the neonate varies from author to author. Using true glucose values investigators have found that most infants are asymptomatic until the level falls below 30 mg./100 ml. Most investigators, therefore, consider values of 30 mg./100 ml. or above to be normal in the first 72 hours of life. Values below 30 mg./100 ml. up to 72 hours and below 40 mg./100 ml. thereafter are considered to be hypoglycemic. In a series of 35 normal neonates examined by Guthrie, Van Leeuwen and Glenn, only two infants had values below 30 mg./100 ml., and both were asymptomatic. One infant had persistent values below 30 mg./100 ml. and one value of 17 mg./100 ml. This infant weighed 2,900 Gm. and was considered normal; but in retrospect its normality can be questioned: on follow-up all of these infants were neurologically normal except that particular infant, whose I.Q. was in the low-normal range and was lower than the I.Q. of his siblings at comparable ages. The child had no motor deficits, however.

LOW-BIRTHWEIGHT AND OTHER HIGH-RISK INFANTS

In the low-birthweight infant, blood sugar values tend to be lower than those seen in full-term infants. Extensive studies by Ward, Baens et al. and Cornblath et al. have indicated mean sugar values of 47 mg./100 ml. at 0-6 hours, 41 mg./100 ml. at 36 hours and 50 mg./100 ml. at 48 hours, as well as many values below 30 mg./100 ml. (15-20%) in low-birthweight infants. Studies by Guthrie et al. of 109 low-birthweight and other high-risk infants showed a high percentage with low blood sugars: 7.3% had at least two blood glucose determinations below 20 mg./100 ml. and 18.4% had at least one determination below 20 mg./100 ml. Of 38 low-birthweight infants in this study, 13% had two or more values below 20 mg./100 ml. and 50% had at least one value below 20 mg./100 ml. None of these infants had symptoms of hypoglycemia at any time during the first 4 days of life (the period of the study). An additional 15 patients—5.2% of the total—had symptomatic hypoglycemia. This compares favorably with an incidence of 5.7% symptomatic hypoglycemia in a series reported by Cornblath.

After feedings are initiated, blood sugar levels tend to rise; however, the rise is less striking than that seen in normal term infants. Blood sugars may remain significantly lower in low-birthweight infants for as long as 1 month after birth.

What, then, constitutes hypoglycemia? Because blood sugars below 30 mg./100 ml. in the term infant are rare and tend to be transient, this level has been chosen as the arbitrary cutoff point in term infants. Because values as low as 20 mg./100 ml. are reasonably common in high-risk infants, including those of low birthweight and premature birth, this value has been chosen as the lower limit of normal by several authors. Values below 30 mg./100 ml. in the term infant or below 20 mg./100 ml. in the low-birthweight or high-risk infant are called hypoglycemic. These figures are based on statistical frequency, however—not upon an evaluation of effect. Inasmuch as there is no convincing evidence as yet that the high-risk infant is less susceptible to the damaging effect of a low blood sugar than is the term infant, we have chosen in our nursery to define as hypoglycemic all values below 30 mg./100 ml. in all infants. The validity of this belief remains to be substantiated or refuted by long-term follow-up of infants with and without low blood sugars. Until proof exists, we feel the infant should be given the benefit of the doubt and treatment initiated to prevent the blood glucose level from dropping below 30 mg./100 ml. We use that value as the indicator for initiating treatment irrespective of the presence or absence of symptoms of hypoglycemia, because infants frequently have values below 20 mg./100 ml. without symptoms.

CLINICAL PICTURE OF HYPOGLYCEMIA

A variety of infants should be watched closely for symptomatic or asymptomatic hypoglycemia. Among these are infants of diabetic or toxemic mothers, infants with erythroblastosis fetalis or polycythemia, the asphyxiated infant, the smaller of twins, the small-for-gestational-age infant, all premature infants and any infant subjected to intrauterine or extrauterine stress.

The infants may present a variety of symptoms and signs—or none at all. As indicated by the series of Guthrie et al., asymptomatic hypoglycemia occurs far more frequently than symptomatic hypoglycemia. Symptoms that have been reported include those listed in Table 9-2. Many of the signs are nonspecific. Apathy and refusal to feed are frequently seen during sepsis. Convulsions are seen with a variety of CNS problems, and jitteriness is seen with hypocalcemia, which may in fact coexist with hypoglycemia. Thus, few of these signs can be considered specific for hypoglycemia; rather, they should serve to alert the clinician to the probability of a sick infant, who should then receive the appropriate physical and laboratory examination to discern the basis of his problem.

In general, hypoglycemia is a problem of the first few hours of life, but it has been reported to occur as late as 7 days of age. It may be recurrent over the first few days of life. We have observed its onset as early as 30 minutes of age in infants of diabetic or toxemic mothers. Hypoglycemia is often more refractory to treatment in the infant of the diabetic or toxemic mother and in infants of very low birthweight for their gestational age.

Prompt diagnosis and treatment is essential, for continued hypoglycemia can result in damage to the central nervous system. In addition, hypoglycemia of 24 hours or more does not respond well to therapy, and response may be delayed for 12-24 hours or may be incomplete. The diagnosis of hypoglycemia is confirmed by determining blood glucose levels in the laboratory, but the Dextrostix may be a valuable screening tool for early detection of low or falling blood sugar levels.

PATHOGENESIS

With the exception of the infant of the diabetic mother, hypoglycemia in the neonate is thought to be due to inadequate stores of meta-

Table 9-2. SYMPTOMATIC HYPOGLYCEMIA IN 56 INFANTS*

Clinical Manifestation	Number of Infants Seen	Number Presenting Sign
Tremors (jitteriness)	42	20
Cyanosis	43	19
Convulsions	29	9
Apnea and irregular respiration	23	6
Apathy	16	2
Cry: high-pitched or weak	10	1
Limpness	13	4
Refusal to feed	5	1
Eye-rolling	2	2
Tachypnea	35	10

*From Cornblath, M., and Schwartz, R.: Disorders of Carbohydrate Metabolism (Philadelphia: W. B. Saunders Company, 1966), p. 88.

bolic substances used by the body in glucose production and to the high glucose requirement of certain organs, notably the brain. In the presence of certain conditions, such as toxemia of pregnancy, placental insufficiency, dysmaturity and prematurity, body stores of glycogen and fat are inadequate; at the same time, the neonate has a high demand for glucose. The brain alone requires 3-5 mg./kg. per minute. The liver's normal net production of glucose is about 3.5 mg./kg. per minute—which is less than adequate to maintain the brain alone. The result of a high utilization rate coupled with inadequate production of glucose is a fall in blood glucose levels. This fall in blood glucose activates the many control mechanisms which are designed to prevent hypoglycemia. There is a release of glucagon, epinephrine, glucocorticoids and growth hormone; these hormones stimulate glycogenolysis, lipolysis and gluconeogenesis. But if glycogen, fat and protein stores are deficient, limited substrate is available for the action of these hormones. Net glucose production goes up only by a limited amount, until the stores are completely exhausted; then glucose levels again fall. In the Guthrie, Van Leeuwen and Glenn series of patients at the University of Missouri this pattern of glucose

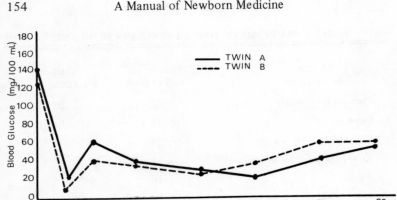

Fig. 9-1.—Blood glucose levels in a set of identical twins.

response was frequently seen in untreated, unfed neonates (Fig. 9-1). There was an initial fall in blood glucose from cord blood levels. This initial fall to hypoglycemic values was followed by an unsustained rise in glucose levels of 20-40 mg./100 ml., then another fall to hypoglycemic levels. The second fall was accompanied by sustained hypoglycemia until feeding or parenteral glucose was initiated. These data do not prove, but do tend to support, the concept that the infant body is trying to correct the hypoglycemia; i.e., we infer that the body recognizes hypoglycemia, even in the asymptomatic neonate, as an undesirable condition.

TREATMENT OF NEONATAL HYPOGLYCEMIA

The blood glucose level of all high-risk infants should be followed at frequent intervals: every 30 minutes for the first 1-2 hours, then every 1-3 hours until fluids or feedings are initiated. This can be done with the Dextrostix alone or more accurately with the Dextrostix-reflectance meter system. Because errors in these methods tend to be on the low side, they will detect more hypoglycemia than actually exists; but this error is to the benefit of the infant. By Dextrostix, values below 30 mg./100 ml. should be investigated and treated. If only the standard Dextrostix scale is available, values below 45 mg./100 ml. can only be inferred and so should be further investigated. When low values are found, a

Hypoglycemia in the Newborn

blood sample is sent to the laboratory for confirmation and therapy is immediately initiated. Blood for calcium determinations is usually drawn simultaneously, because hypocalcemia frequently coexists with hypoglycemia.

Therapy of hypoglycemia consists of 2-3 ml. of 50% glucose diluted to 25% glucose with water for injection, given by slow intravenous push. In the infants of diabetic mothers, push therapy should be avoided because of the glucose stimulation of insulin production, which causes profound hypoglycemia. This initial therapy is followed by a drip of 10-20% glucose in water in a dose of 65-100 ml./kg. per day during the first 48 hours of life and 100-130 ml./kg. per day thereafter. One-fourth N saline can be added after 48-72 hours of life if intravenous doses are to be continued. The intravenous therapy should be withdrawn very slowly, because there is a tendency for the hypoglycemia to recur. Sutherland has shown that the infant's blood sugar is highly dependent on the rate of flow of the fluids. Changes in drip rate will vary the blood sugar from hyper- to hypoglycemic levels. Constant flow rates are therefore highly desirable and can best be attained by infusion pumps. This is especially true when intra-arterial fluids are used through the umbilical artery and administered against a high head of pressure.

If hypoglycemia recurs, in spite of intravenous therapy, additional doses of 50% glucose can be administered; or adrenal steroids may be used. Hydrocortisone is a dose of 5 mg./kg. per day, given twice daily (or an equivalent dose of prednisone, once daily) or ACTH, four units twice daily, is recommended. We have rarely found it necessary to use steroids in our patients with hypoglycemia. Intravenous glucose up to 20% solution has proven effective in 98% of infants, excluding those of diabetic mothers. It should be pointed out, however, that glucose solutions of 15% or more are sclerosing to peripheral veins and that solutions above 20% can be damaging to the liver if umbilical vein catheters are below the liver or in the liver parenchyma. The tip of the artery catheters should not be in the area of ostia of the major abdominal arteries, because stenosis of these vessels may result form the irritation of concentrated solutions.

Except for a transient response, glucagon and epinephrine are relatively ineffective glycemic agents in the majority of hypoglycemic infants because glycogen and fat stores are inadequate. Such agents are more effective in the infant of the diabetic mother; indeed, for this infant they may constitute primary therapy.

PREVENTION

Much has been written about the desirability of early vs. late feeding of neonates and about the desirability of preventing hypoglycemia. There are very limited data, however, to show that hypoglycemia is permanently damaging if not prevented or vigorously treated. Until all the facts are in, one should give the benefit of the doubt to the infant, either by preventing the problem or by recognizing and vigorously treating it when present.

In a study by Beard, prematurely born infants fed early were able to sustain a blood glucose level between feedings at a statistically higher value than infants fed later (Fig. 9-2). By 72 hours the early-fed infants had mean preprandial glucose values of over 50 mg./100 ml. and the late-fed infants had mean values of about 20 mg./100 ml. Similar trends have been found in term infants, but the differences are not so striking. Tests of tolerance for epinephrine, glucagon and combinations of these substances have been made on infants fed early and infants fed late. (Early feedings were at 3-6 hours of age, late feedings at about 12-24 hours of age. The tests were performed at 24-48 hours of age). In all of these tests, early-fed infants responded to these hormonal agents, either alone or in combination, with higher blood glucose levels than did later-fed infants. These data indicate that early-fed infants build and maintain more adequate glycogen reserves than do infants fed later. We infer, then, that unfed infants use what meager glycogen stores they may have to prevent hypoglycemia during the early hours. Even late-fed infants who do not have clinical or laboratory hypoglycemia are, nonetheless, in a more precarious position regarding glycogen reserve than are the early-fed or treated infants.

Beard found that serum bilirubin levels are statistically lower up to 144 hours of life in early-fed vs. late-fed infants. In 34 premature infants the mean bilirubin at 120 hours of age, for instance, was 11 mg./100 ml. in late-fed infants and 7 mg./100 ml. in early-fed infants.

Rabor et al. have shown that the time required to regain birthweight in premature infants is less in early-fed infants than it is in late-fed infants. In a group of 254 premature infants the mean time for regaining

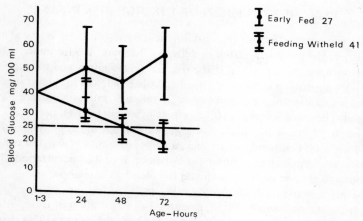

Fig. 9-2.—Blood glucose levels in uncomplicated premature infants.

birthweight was 9 days in 87 infants fed at 6 hours, 11 days in 33 infants fed at 12 hours, and 15 days in 137 infants fed at 24 hours. There was also a higher mortality in the late-fed infants in all weight groups. At all weights except 1,250-1,500 Gm. nasogastric feeding early did not decrease the mortality, but early intravenous feeding did decrease the mortality. The differences here were most marked in infants weighing 765-1,001 Gm.

Data on the neurologic status of symptomatic hypoglycemic infants are limited, and almost no data are available on asymptomatic infants. In Ward's series 10% of hypoglycemic infants were dead on follow-up and 20% showed obvious mental and neurologic defects. In a study by Zetterstom 50% of infants with hypoglycemia were found, on follow-up, to have epilepsy. All these infants had symptomatic hypo-glycemia which presented as convulsions; these children, therefore, may have had some underlying brain defect.

Everyone who has treated infants with hypoglycemia has had the experience of seeing many of them develop normally. Such infants usually had an early diagnosis and prompt, vigorous treatment. Altogether, it seems reasonable to conclude that prevention or prompt, vigorous treatment of hypoglycemia in high-risk infants will promote his survival and well-being, as measured by a variety of clinical and biochemical parameters.

PLAN OF TREATMENT OF THE HIGH-RISK INFANT

In our nursery, when a high-risk infant is born or if there is any abnormality in the pregnancy, labor or delivery, the infant is kept under close observation in an incubator. If the risk factors are minor and the infant appears normal, he is simply warmed and observed, and his blood sugar level is measured by Dextrostix every 30 minutes until feedings are begun. The usual feeding is 10% dextrose in water (D10W), begun at ½-1 hour of age. If the infant is reasonably well but moderately is small (2,000-2,500 Gm.) and cannot suck, a nasogastric tube is inserted and D10W is administered, beginning at ½-1 hour. If oral administration of fluids and glucose does not maintain the blood glucose above 40 mg./100 ml., parenteral administration is begun.

If the infant is small or is ill, parenteral administration of fluids is begun immediately upon his admission to the high-risk nursery. This may be done through a peripheral vein or through the umbilical artery or vein. In our nursery we prefer a peripheral vein or the umbilical artery. If the umbilical vein is to be used, careful placement by radiography must be carried out to be sure the catheter is through the liver and into the inferior vena cava, to avoid damage to the liver. Umbilical artery placement should be away from the ostia of the major abdominal vessels. D10W is begun at the rate of 60-65 ml./kg. per day; and the blood glucose is monitored. If blood glucose falls below 40 mg./100 ml. by Dextrostix, the rate of administration or the concentration of glucose, or both, is increased. Small doses of 50% glucose are administered as needed. The volume of fluids is increased daily to 150 mg./kg. per day according to the usual values of fluid administered in newborns.

With this therapy, blood glucose levels rarely fall below 60 mg./100 ml. and are usually in the range of 90-100 mg./100 ml. Steroids or other hormonal agents are seldom used in our nursery for treatment of hypoglycemic infants. Steroids or epinephrine are sometimes needed in infants of diabetic mothers, but most other high-risk infants benefit from glucose administration to correct the specific deficiency. If the infant is refractory to simple glucose administration, other diseases, such as diabetes in the mother, glycogen storage disease and other inborn errors of metabolism, should be ruled out.

Small-for-gestational-age infants and polycythemic infants have a more refractory hypoglycemia. Postmature or dysmature infants frequently have extremely depleted glycogen and fat stores, and the physician commonly underestimates the quantity of glucose required to maintain them. Because their reserves are poor, their response to hormones as well as to steroids is reduced. We have often found it necessary to use 20% glucose solutions, with frequent doses of 50% glucose, to maintain these infants.

Polycythemic infants with refractory hypoglycemia are best treated by removal of the excess red blood cells and by facilitating the circulation. Red blood cells may be removed by simple phlebotomy and fluid administration, in mild cases, or by exchange transfusion with lower hematocrit blood, in more severe cases. Hypoglycemia is frequently self-correcting with correction of the hematocrit, but glucose administration is nonetheless indicated.

Erythroblastosis fetalis is sometimes accompanied by hypoglycemia. This problem is thought to be due to hyperinsulinemia. In severely affected patients, hypoglycemia should be watched for before, during and after exchange transfusion. Treatment should be initiated immediately if a falling blood glucose is found.

A variety of other hypoglycemic conditions have been described, but they are so rare that they need not be described here. Rather, this discussion has been intended to describe the problems of glucose homeostasis in the commonly encountered high-risk infant and to outline the methods currently recommended for prevention, recognition and treatment of this common problem.

SUGGESTED READINGS

1. Adamson, K., Jr.: Transport of Organic Substances and Oxygen across the Placenta, in Bergsma, D. (ed.): *Symposium on the Placenta,* National Foundation, Birth Defects Orig. Art. Ser. 1:27, 1965.
2. Baens, G. S., Lundeen, E., and Cornblath, M.: Studies of carbohydrate metabolism in the newborn infant. VI. Levels of glucose in blood in premature infants, Pediatrics 31:580, 1963.
3. Baens, G. S., Lundeen E., and Cornblath, M.: Studies of carbohydrate metabolism in the newborn infants. VI. Levels of glucose in blood in premature infants, Pediatrics 31:580, 1963.

4. Beard, A. G., Panos, T. C., Marasigan, G. U., Emenians, J., Kennedy, H. F., and Lamb, J.: Perinatal stress and the premature neonate. II. Effect of fluid and calorie deprivation on blood glucose, J. Pediat. 68:359, 1966.

5. Cornblath, M., and Schwartz, R.: *Disorders of Carbohydrate Metabolism* (Philadelphia: W. B. Saunders Company, 1966), p. 34.

6. Cornblath, M., Ganzon, A. F., Nicolopaulas, D., Baens, G., Hollander, R. J., Gordon, M. H., and Gordon, H. H.: Studies of carbohydrate metabolism in the newborn infant. III. Some factors influencing the capillary blood sugar and the response to glucagon during the first hours of life, Pediatrics 27:378, 1961.

7. Cornblath, M., and Reesner, S. H.: Blood glucose in the neonate and its clinical significance, New England J. Med. 273:278, 1965.

8. Cornblath, M., Wyhregt, S. H., and Baens, G. S.: Studies of carbohydrate metabolism in the newborn infant. VII. Levels of glucose in blood in premature infants, Pediatrics 31:580, 1963.

9. Cornblath, M., O'Dell, G. B., and Levin, E. Y.: Symptomatic neonatal hypoglycemia associated with toxemia of pregnancy, J. Pediat. 55:545, 1959.

10. Cornblath, M., Wyhregt, S. H., and Baens, G. S.: Studies of carbohydrate metabolism in the newborn infant. VII. Tests of carbohydrate tolerance in premature infants, Pediatrics 32:1007, 1963.

11. Creery, R. D. G., and Parkinson, T. J.: Blood glucose changes in the newborn. I. The blood glucose pattern of normal infants in the first 12 hours of life, Arch. Dis. Childhood 28:134, 1953.

12. Farquhar, J. W.: Control of the blood sugar level in the neonatal period, Arch. Dis. Childhood 29:519, 1954.

13. From, G. A., Driscoll, S. G., and Steinke, J.: Serum insulin in newborn infants with erythroblastosis fetalis, Pediatrics 44:549, 1969.

14. Gandy, G. M., Adamson, K., Cunningham, N., Silverman, W. A., and James, L.S.: Thermal environment and acid-base homeostasis in human infants during the first few hours of life, J. Clin. Invest. 43:751, 1964.

15. Guthrie, R. A., Van Leeuwen, G., and Glenn, L.: The frequency of asymptomatic hypoglycemia in the high-risk newborn infant, Pediatrics 46:933, 1970.

16. Humbert, H. R., Abelson, H., Hathaway, W. E., and Battaglia, F.: Polycythemia in small for gestational age infants, J. Pediat. 75:812, 1969.

17. James, E. J., Raye, J. R., Gresham, E. L., Makowski, E. L., Meschia, G., and Battaglia, F. D.: The normal oxygen consumption and respiratory quotient of the mammalian fetus, Pediat. Res. 5:497, 1971.

18. Lamb, J., Beard, A. G., and Panos, T. G.: Relationships between plasma free acids, glucose and bilirubin values in the neonate, Proc. Sc. Soc. Pediat. Res. 1963 (abst.).
19. McCann, M. L., and Burr, D.: Ames Reflectance Meter/Dextrostix System—A New Screening Test for the Detection of Neonatal Hypoglycemia, in *Ames Laboratories Compendium on the Use of the Reflectance Meter,* 1970.
20. McCann, M. L., Miyazaki, Y., Guthrie, R. A., and Jackson, R. L.: A new therapeutic rationale for the infant of the diabetic mother, Missouri Med. 65:275, 1968.
21. Mulligan, P. B., and Schwartz, R.: Hepatic carbohydrate metabolism in the genesis of neonatal hypoglycemia, Pediatrics 30:125, 1962.
22. Norval, M. A., Kennedy, R. L. J., and Berkson, J.: Blood sugar in newborn infants. J. Pediat. 34:342, 1949.
23. Rabor, I. F., Oh, W., Wu, P. Y. K., Metcalf, J., Vaughn, M. A. O., and Gobler, M: The effects of early and late feeding of intrauterine fetally malnourished (IUM) infants, Pediatrics 42:261, 1968.
24. Somogyi, M.: Determination of blood sugar, J. Biol. Chem. 160:69, 1965.
25. Teller, J. D.: Direct quantitive, colorimetric determination serum or plasma glucose (abst.), in Proc. 130th Meeting Am. Chem. Soc., 1956, p. 690.
26. Ward, O. C: Blood sugar studies on premature babies, Arch. Dis. Childhood 28:194, 1953.
27. Widdas, W. F.: Transport mechanism in the foetus, Brit. M. Bull. 17:107, 1961.
28. Zetterstom, R.: Discussing neonatal hypoglycemia, Ann. New York Acad. Sc. 111:537, 1963.

CHAPTER 10

Infants of Diabetic Mothers and Transient Hyperglycemia

G. VAN LEEUWEN, M.D.

Y. MIYAZAKI, M.D.

INFANTS OF DIABETIC MOTHERS

In 1959, Gellis wrote a comprehensive review of the problems facing the physician who provides care for the infant of the diabetic mother. He reported that 35% of conceptions in diabetic women end in death by abortion, intrauterine death or neonatal death. No more recent mortality data are available, but we believe that the mortality is significantly lower, for a number of reasons: improved control of the diabetes; improved diagnosis of the proper time for delivery, by means of placental function tests; and advanced neonatal care. Of equal importance is the fact that, because of more sophisticated neonatal care, the morbidity and subsequent brain damage has probably been reduced. This chapter discusses the problems encountered by infants of the diabetic mother and presents an acceptable method of treating these problems.

Attention to meticulous detail in managing the diabetic woman during pregnancy, and particularly during the last trimester, can significantly lessen the problems of the baby. One internist-diabetologist has recommended that pregnant diabetics be confined to bed during the last trimester, have a controlled diet and exercise, and take four injections of regular insulin daily, to assure good control. This approach is not economically feasible at this time, but the concept is sound; one should come as close to it as possible, maintaining control so that a 1+ glycosuria is the most that is acceptable.

In addition to the excellent control, an anesthesiologist and a pediatrician should be advised of impending delivery, both to instill calmness in the family and to be properly prepared.

Delivery should be accomplished as near 38 weeks' gestation as possible, or earlier if urinary estriol levels are dangerously low. The pediatrician should be alerted as soon as the decision has been made to induce labor.

Symptoms and Treatment

To promote a better understanding of the problems of the infant of the diabetic mother, we have classified the problems in two groups: the "killers" and the "spoilers."

A summary of all the possible abnormal findings in infants of diabetic mothers is presented in Table 10-1. A typical infant, showing cushingoid appearance, obesity and lethargy, is pictured in Figure 10-1.

Death in the liveborn infant of the diabetic mother is usually due to hyaline membrane syndrome or to serious congenital malformations. The rapid and correct diagnosis of hyaline membrane syndrome is described in Chapter 5, on respiratory disorders. The time of onset, symptoms and treatment are identical with those of the high-risk, low-birthweight baby

Congenital malformations of a serious or lethal nature occur in some 10-15% of infants of diabetic mothers. The most common serious malformation is cyanotic congenital heart disease. We have encountered the

Table 10-1. PROBLEMS OF THE INFANT OF THE DIABETIC MOTHER

Congenital anomalies in 10-15% of infants

Respiratory distress syndrome

Prematurity

Jaundice

Hypocalcemic tetany

Plethora and polycythemia

Poor feeding

Increased susceptibility to infection

Increased neurologic deficiency and behavior problems

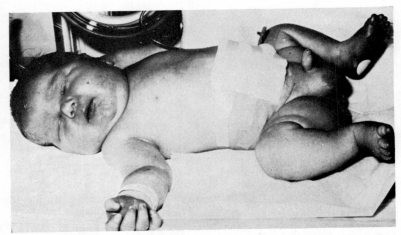

Fig. 10-1.—Typical appearance of a sick infant of a diabetic mother. Note the cushingoid appearance and the floppy, expressionless and sleepy characteristics. An umbilical artery catheter is in place. This appearance has prompted a saying about these babies: "Some of us are out of breath, many of us are ugly, and all of us are fat."

entire spectrum of anomalies, including phocomelia, meningomyelocele, anencephaly and tracheal cyst, in infants of diabetic mothers.

During a recent year two of our infants died primarily as a result of disseminated intravascular coagulation (DIC). One of the infants had hyaline membrane syndrome; the other seemed normal except for some hypoglycemia. Both mothers were severe diabetics (juvenile onset) but had been in reasonably good control and had had good prenatal care. We are unable to explain why these infants had DIC; however, this entity may have excaped our attention in earlier years. Both babies failed to respond to heparin therapy.

Infants of diabetic mothers seem particularly susceptible to neonatal septicemia (discussed in Chapter 8).

The triad of hypoglycemia, hypocalcemia, and hyperbilirubinemia in infants of diabetic mothers is well known. Since we have learned to either prevent or treat the hypoglycemia early, we have had a considerably lower incidence of tetany and jaundice.

Jaundice usually begins on the second or third day. It seems to be an exaggerated "physiologic" jaundice and may be due to glucuronyl transferase deficiency. In past years a significant percentage of these infants have required exchange transfusion, but now phototherapy is used when the indirect bilirubin exceeds 10 mg./100 ml. This has essentially eliminated the need for exchange transfusion.

Hypocalcemic tetany likewise has decreased in frequency since we have learned to prevent hypoglycemia, although when it occurs it is particularly resistant to therapy. We believe that tetany is more common when glucagon is used to treat the hypoglycemia, but this has not been documented. When tetany occurs it usually responds to 10% calcium gluconate, 1 ml./kg. intravascularly; this dose may be repeated as often as necessary to return calcium levels to normal. These small doses usually do not produce bradycardia when given slowly. After symptoms have subsided, calcium gluconate or lactate is added to the formula intake in amounts equal to the total daily dose which was required parenterally.

Abnormal glucose metabolism is the most common abnormality in infants of diabetic mothers and is present to some degree in most infants. Infants can be divided into groups (Table 10-2) according to whether too much, too little or the correct amount of insulin is produced. If the mother is hyperglycemic the fetus is hyperglycemic, because glucose readily crosses the placental membrane. The fetal pancreas responds by producing excessive insulin. After delivery the baby, deprived of glucose from the mother, is hyperinsulinemic; correlatively it is also hypoglycemic in accordance with the degree of hyperinsulinism. It follows that in some instances (two of 40 cases, in one report)

Table 10-2. VARIATIONS IN GLUCOSE METABOLISM AND APPROPRIATE THERAPY, IN INFANTS OF DIABETIC MOTHERS

Proportion of Infants	Clinical Findings	Therapy
Most	Minimal hypoglycemia	Glucose orally, early
Some	Normal	Glucose orally, early
Some	Refractory hypoglycemia	Glucose parenterally; cortisone; epinephrine (?)
Few	Hyperglycemia	Insulin?

the fetus who will himself one day become diabetic may exhaust his pancreas because of excessive work and may possibly develop a diabetic acidosis-like state with hyperglycemia after birth. It has been suggested but not documented that the high rate of intrauterine death at about 38 weeks' gestation may be due to this diabetic-like state.

The baby may have normal glucose levels if the mother is well controlled. Most will have some hypoglycemia, nearly always during the first 3 hours of life. Some will have severe and refractory hypoglycemia. An occasional infant may develop a diabetic-like state; we have not had an opportunity to treat such infants with insulin, but we presume that they would respond to this therapy. Transient diabetes or transient neonatal hyperglycemia appears to be unrelated to diabetes; however, it is most conveniently discussed at the end of this chapter. Beckwith's syndrome, or visceral organomegaly with hypoglycemia, is also unrelated to diabetes.

There is some evidence indicating that mothers who are well controlled with respect to their diabetes before and during pregnancy and labor will give birth to the most nearly normal infants. If the mother has received adequate insulin therapy, the baby need produce only enough for his own needs. But too many internists and obstetricians are content with "reasonable" control, when really good control might greatly enhance the baby's chance to be normal.

Our treatment of the infant of the diabetic mother is direct and simple. The Dextrostix test is done at birth and every 30 minutes thereafter until the threat of hypoglycemia has passed. If the blood glucose begins to drop rapidly during the first hour, as is usually the case, 10% glucose in water is given—by nipple if tolerated, otherwise by gavage, 30-60 ml. each hour. If hypoglycemia develops in spite of this, an umbilical artery is catheterized and glucose is given intravascularly, 1 Gm./kg. in a solution of 20 Gm./100 ml. This is followed by a 10% glucose water drip, 60-90 ml./kg. per day. Other agents, such as sodium bicarbonate or calcium gluconate, may be added to this solution as indicated. Oral feedings are introduced as soon as tolerated, and parenteral administration of fluids is discontinued as soon as normoglycemia is easily maintained.

A word of caution about the above therapy is indicated. Ten percent glucose is a hypertonic solution. It will sclerose peripheral veins—which is of no great consequence. However, when it is injected into the liver via the umbilical vein, it is likely to cause significant damage. We avoid the administration of any hypertonic solutions into an umbilical vein unless x-ray has shown us that the catheter is in the vena cava or right atrium, above the diaphragm. Hypertonic solutions should always be given into the largest possible vessel, to facilitate rapid dilution.

One must also avoid obtaining blood glucose levels from blood withdrawn from umbilical catheters. This will result in artefactually high levels, because glucose is being administered into the same catheter.

We have recently reported on the indications for epinephrine therapy in infants with refractory hypoglycemia. We concluded that the use of subcutaneous epinephrine is indicated only in infants who develop rapid hypoglycemia following a therapeutic dose of glucose (1 Gm./kg.) intravascularly. By the type of response the baby can be clinically judged to have hyperinsulinism. That situation seems to arise most often in the poorly controlled gestational or insulin-dependent diabetic. When used, epinephrine should be given in a dose of 50 μg./kg. as Susphrine, diluted 10 times with saline. Although we are now studying the infants in less depth, we continue to make two observations: (1) that mothers who have had good control seldom have infants who suffer from refractory hypoglycemia and (2) that the administration of epinephrine is rarely necessary, although it is very effective when administered for the proper reason.

Even though we give these infants vigorous attention almost from the moment of birth, we continue to encounter some who have been metabolically corrected but still have a protracted morbidity. This is usually prolonged acidosis, respiratory distress or anorexia. We cannot explain why this occurs—except that, again, they are infants of poorly controlled diabetics. Presumably, if their glucose, calcium, bilirubin, pH and oxygen tension are maintained in the normal range, permanent brain damage can be prevented.

It is important to remember that it is easy to overlook one of these babies until damage has been done. It is, of course, simple to make the diagnosis "infant of a diabetic"; but if the mother is prediabetic or has not been recognized as a gestational diabetic, the diagnosis is difficult. Infants of prediabetic mothers have all the familiar problems, although not as intensely. Careful observation of all infants who weigh over 9 pounds helps to detect some of these infants, but not all. We find our transitional nursery, in which all newborn infants are placed for 24 hours, is particularly useful in these cases, because here the nurses perform frequent Dextrostix tests (along with other monitoring). We have now collected histories of a small group of infants, weighing 8-9 pounds, in whose mothers diabetes was not suspected but yet there was early hypoglycemia. These mothers have either remembered a relative with diabetes or have themselves had an abnormal glucose tolerance test.

Prognosis

Mortality in liveborn infants of diabetics is very low but is, nevertheless, a factor. On our service two of the last 25 such infants have died—one with a lethal anomaly and one with disseminated intravascular coagulation.

Summary

The infant of the diabetic mother is subject to all the problems of other risk infants and is most likely to have some of them. Careful monitoring, early treatment of hyaline membrane syndrome, vigorous treatment of nonlethal anomalies, maintaining normal pH and P_{O_2} supporting the baby with glucose and calcium if necessary, and control of the serum bilirubin constitute the core of the treatment. Mortality has thus been decreased and morbidity significantly lessened.

TRANSIENT DIABETES MELLITUS IN EARLY INFANCY

It is difficult to find an appropriate place in this book for a discussion of transient diabetes mellitus in infancy, because this condition does not necessarily occur in infants of diabetic mothers. We have encountered this syndrome with increasing frequency, possibly because we have been searching for it more intensively. Infants with this condition are not to be confused with a number of small-risk infants who have received considerable amounts of 10% glucose during their acute stages and who develop a progressive hyperglycemia during this period. The latter are simply experiencing a glucose overload, which of course is not related to the syndrome of transient diabetes, or transient hyperglycemia.

Hyperglycemia in the newborn may be identified as a blood glucose level greater than 125 mg./100 ml. after a 4-hour fast. From practical experience, infants who have this syndrome have blood glucose levels greatly in excess of this. Not many infants with this condition have been reported. In Cornblath's review a total of 15 patients were identified. Many other patients are known to us, however—the frequency being such that individual patients are no longer being presented.

The clinical manifestations are hyperglycemia, glycosuria, dehydration (which may be severe) and absence of ketonuria. All of the infants are of low birthweight, although many are full term. The sexes are equally represented. The most striking sign usually is marked dehydration and wasting. The signs probably will not cause physicians to suspect transient diabetes, but frequent Dextrostix monitoring of the blood sugar of the sick infant will suggest this diagnosis. The diagnosis then is based on glycosuria or hyperglycemia. The highest blood glucose level we have seen is 800 mg./100 ml. We have now cared for six patients with this disorder; two died. One of those who died had been given insulin.

Some of the patients do not require insulin. Those who do, respond rather dramatically to it. We use 1-3 units per kilogram of body weight per day, for periods ranging from a few days to as long as a year, the duration of this illness being extremely variable. We rehydrate the infant with 5% glucose; give appropriate sodium bicarbonate to correct the acidosis; and switch to oral feedings as quickly as possible. We prescribe a regular infant diet for the infant.

One must keep in mind that permanent diabetes mellitus has been reported in the neonate, and one should not be totally surprised if the infant does not completely recover from the above-outlined therapy. Of the four patients who recovered, all have repeatedly shown normal tolerance for glucose, orally and intravenously, up to 3 years of age (the longest time we have followed any of our patients). Some physicians prefer not to include any glucose in the initial fluids; instead, they simply use a hypotonic saline solution at the rate of 60-80 ml./kg. Once the blood sugar has fallen below 300 mg./100 ml., fluids can be increased to 150-200 ml./kg. per day. Because of the extreme sensitivity of some patients to insulin, we prefer using 5% glucose in the initial fluids.

We do not as yet understand the etiology of this syndrome. We suspect that these may be infants who will eventually become diabetic, but to date this has not been documented. The prognosis for those infants who survive appears to be excellent: our four infants, followed up to age 3 years, are normal.

SUGGESTED READINGS

1. Burland, W. L.: Diabetes mellitus syndrome in the newborn infant, J. Pediat. 65:122, 1964.
2. Cordero, L. J., et al.: Fetal response to glucose infusion: How much credit does the fetal pancreas deserve? Pediatrics 46:155, 1970.
3. Cornblath, M., et al.: Infants of the diabetic mother, Advances Metab. Dis. (suppl.) 1:2414, 1970.
4. Cornblath, M., and Schwartz, R.: *Disorders of Carbohydrate Metabolism in Infancy* (Philadelphia: W. B. Saunders Company, 1966).
5. Driscoll, S. G., Benirschke, K., and Curtis, G. W.: Neonatal deaths among infants of diabetic mothers, Am. J. Dis. Child. 100:818, 1960.
6. Farquhar, J. W.: The infant of diabetic mother, Postgrad. M. J. suppl. 8064, 1969.
7. Farquhar, J. W.: Prognosis for babies born to diabetic mothers in Edinburgh, Arch. Dis. Childhood 44:233, 1969.
8. Farquhar, J. W.: The child of the diabetic woman, Arch. Dis. Childhood 34:76, 1959.
9. Gerrard, J. W., and Chin, W.: The syndrome of transient diabetes, J. Pediat. 61:89, 1962.
10. Greenwood, R., and Traisman, H.: Permanent diabetes mellitus in a neonate, J. Pediat. 79:296, 1971.
11. Hagbard, L.: *Pregnancy and Diabetes Mellitus* (Springfield, Ill.: Charles C Thomas, Publisher, 1961).
12. Hagbard, L., Olow, I., and Reinarid, T.: Follow-up study of 514 children of diabetic mothers, Acta paediat. 48:184, 1959.
13. Keidan, S. E.: Transient diabetes in infancy, Arch. Dis. Childhood 30:291, 1955.
14. King, K. C., et al.: Infants of diabetic mothers, Pediatrics 45:889, 1970.
15. Long, W. N., et al.: Diabetes and pregnancy, Johns Hopkins Med. J. suppl. 8064, 1969.
16. McCann, M. I.: Infants of diabetic mothers, Pediatrics 45:887, 1970.
17. Navarrete, V. N., et al.: The significance of metabolic adjustment before a new pregnancy. Prophylaxis of congenital malformations, Am. J. Obst. & Gynec. 107:250, 1970.

18. Pedersen, J.: *The Pregnant Diabetic and Her Newborn: Problems and Management* (Baltimore: The Williams & Wilkins Co., 1967).
19. Pedersen, L. M., Tygstrup, D., and Pedersen, J.: Congenital malformations in newborn infants of diabetic women. Correlation with maternal vascular complications, Lancet 1:1124, 1964.
20. Rubins, A., and Murphy, D. P.: Studies in human reproduction. III. The frequency of congenital malformations in the offspring of non-diabetic and diabetic individuals, J. Pediat. 53:579, 1958.
21. Wolf, J., et al.: The influence of maternal glucose infections on fetal growth hormone levels, Pediatrics 45:36, 1970.

CHAPTER 11

Congenital Heart Disease

PAUL MOORING, M.D.

The most important problem, by far, for physicians dealing with babies is to recognize the sick baby. Especially in dealing with disorders of the cardiovascular system, it frequently takes an astute clinician indeed to recognize the subtle early signs of trouble. Most cardiovascular diseases, if detected early, can now be helped greatly by proper medicines and by palliative or curative surgery.

Most of the significant cardiovascular defects in infancy produce either heart murmurs or cyanosis, which alert the physician to the possible presence of a heart defect. One would think this would make detection of heart defects in early life relatively easy. Unfortunately, this is not the case. It is well known that many physicians have difficulty detecting murmurs which are not very loud. This problem is compounded in the baby because of the fast heart rate and the small chest, which makes auscultation difficult; furthermore, there is the handicap of the inadequate stethoscope (long tubing and rubber-tipped stethoscope head) found in most nurseries. The problem of cyanosis is compounded by the common presence of acrocyanosis (cyanosis of the extremities) in normal newborns. The usual lighting in nurseries does not make detection of slight cyanosis of mucous membranes easy.

These special problems will be discussed further in this chapter, which is devoted chiefly to practical aspects of heart disease in the newborn from the viewpoint of the primary physician; i.e., the physician working with infants in the first few weeks of life. He can expect to encounter heart defects in about one of every 140 births. The death rate in these infants is high: one third will die in the first month.

CARDIOVASCULAR EXAMINATION OF THE NEONATE

Preliminary Data

The most important aspect of examining the cardiovascular system of the very young infant is to obtain as much information as possible before disturbing the baby.

Some of the most useful information can be obtained from the nurses' notes and directly from the nurses. If the infant is old enough to eat, find out all about his feeding habits. Is the baby a vigorous eater? Does he appear to tire easily? Check with the nurse to find out whether any cyanosis has been noted.

Check the pattern of heart rate and respiratory rate, from the chart. The average heart rate is 120-130/minute for the first week or two. Respiratory rates average less than 45 in full-term infants and less than 60 in premature infants. Rates consistently above these should arouse suspicion.

Gross Inspection

A great deal can be told by gross inspection of the infant. Probably he is almost nude; if not, do a preliminary examination before undressing him. Spend a minute or two watching the baby. What is his color like? If cyanosis is noted, is it generalized? Does it involve only the hands and feet? Or does it only involve the upper extremities?

Is the baby restless and irritable, or comfortable? What is his breathing pattern? Is his breathing rapid and shallow (tachypnea)? Or is it deep, with retractions (dyspnea)?

Can any gross physical defects be detected? Is the face normal? Are the hands, feet and ears normal or abnormal? Could this be a trisomy condition, Marfan's syndrome, Turner's syndrome or some other chromosomal aberration?

Next, the examiner should feel the pedal pulses (with warm hands). Feeling these most distal pulses is usually easily done—and can be very rewarding. Ordinarily, pedal pulses are easily felt but are not prominent. Bounding pulses would support the diagnosis of patent ductus arteriosus or some less common arterial-venous runoff. Absent pedal pulses in the presence of palpable radial pulses would suggest a coarctation.

Decreased pedal and radial pulses—all of which are difficult to feel—
would suggest possible heart failure with a poor cardiac output or obstruction to outflow from the left ventricle.

After evaluating the pedal pulses, the next least disturbing part of the
examination is to determine liver size and location. A note of warning
here: if the infant has just eaten, use extreme care. Too-forceful palpation after feeding can lead to regurgitation and possible aspiration (a
common cause of death in weakened infants. The liver edge usually is
felt less than 3 cm. (1.5 to 2.5 finger breadths) below the anterior axillary line. A liver edge further than 3 cm. can be a sign of congestive failure, hematologic disorder, liver disorder or depressed diaphragm. The
liver edge in heart failure is usually quite firm and frequently tender.

After palpating the abdomen, the examiner is ready to examine the
chest. As gently as possible, with warm hands, the precordium should
be palpated to (1) determine the presence of thrills and (2) determine
whether or not the precordium is hyperdynamic. The point of maximum
intensity (PMI) should be located; in infants this is normally at the lower
left sternal border. If a thrill is located, note the area where the thrill is
maximum.

If the baby is still resting quietly he can now be auscultated. Preferably the examiner uses his own stethoscope—one whose earpieces fit
snugly. The stethoscope head should be warm. It should have at least a
bell and diaphragm. The tubing should be double, thick and as short as
possible for comfortably reaching the chest. The rubber-tipped stetho-
scopes with 4-foot tubing should never be used: most of the important
sounds will be lost with such an apparatus.

By auscultation the examiner is trying to determine: Is there a murmur? If so, where is it maximum? Is it grade 1, 2, 3 or 4 (on the scale of
6)? Is it harsh, rough, blowing or vibratory? Is the murmur short, holosystolic, crescendo, decrescendo, systolic or (rarely in infants) diastolic?
Where does the murmur transmit to? Is it heard posteriorly?

What is the pulmonic second sound like? Is it single or double? Does
it have a variable or a fixed split? Is it decreased, increased or normal in
intensity?

The lung fields should also be auscultated. The presence of rales most
often indicates infection but may indicate left heart failure.

After all this information is obtained, if the child was not completely
undressed, this can now be done and the examination repeated.

By now the baby is probably crying— and this gives the examiner an opportunity to observe the skin color with exertion. Does the baby get redder or pinker? Or cyanotic?

Because of the rapidly changing hemodynamic status of babies, especially those with heart defects, a single look is frequently misleading or inadequate. A repeat exam in a few hours, or a day or two later, can sometimes help clarify a difficult problem.

THE MOST COMMON HEART DEFECTS OF INFANCY

Classification of Heart Defects

For diagnostic purposes, and to some extent for treatment purposes, it is convenient to divide congenital heart defects into two main and four secondary classes. This classification is based on the presence or absence of cyanosis and the appearance of pulmonary circulation on chest x-rays. The commonest conditions are starred (*).

Acyanotic

Normal pulmonary circulation

Pulmonary stenosis*
Aortic stenosis*
Coarctation*
Idiopathic hypertrophic subaortic stenosis
Mitral stenosis
Endocardial fibroelastosis

Increased pulmonary circulation

Patent ductus arteriosus*
Atrial septal defect*
Ventricular septal defect*
Endocardial cushion defect
Truncus arteriosus
Aorticopulmonary window

Cyanotic

Normal or decreased pulmonary circulation

Tetralogy of Fallot*
Tricuspid atresia
Ebstein's anomaly

Increased pulmonary circulation

Transposition of the great vessels*
Hypoplastic left heart syndrome*
Total anomalous pulmonary vein
Single ventricle

Nine of these lesions are relatively common: altogether they account
for 85-90% of all congenital heart defects. If the primary physician is
reasonably familiar with the characteristics of these nine, this will usually be adequate for treatment purposes. In a recent classification of
heart disease seen in 1,500 infants during the first year of life, cyanotic
heart disease accounted for about 40% and acyanotic heart disease accounted for about 60%.

These different types of defects characteristically bring difficulties
at different ages. In the first week of life the defect most likely to cause
heart failure and cyanosis is the hypoplastic left heart syndrome. After
the second week most infants with this defect have died. Transposition
of the great vessels is the most common cause of cyanosis and heart failure after the first week and for the first few months of life. Coarctation
of the aorta is the most common cause of congestive failure without
cyanosis in the latter part of the first month of life and should be particularly suspected in that age group. The two major left-to-right shunts,
ventricular septal defect and patent ductus arteriosus, usually begin to
cause a lot of trouble after a couple of weeks of age, as pulmonary resistance drops.

For review purposes, what follows is a brief summary of the chief
characteristics of these common defects.

Left-to-Right Shunts

Ventricular septal defects, as isolated heart defects, are the most
common of all heart defects: they account for 22% of all congenital
heart defects as isolated lesions, and they also frequently occur with
other defects (tetralogy of Fallot, transposition of the great vessels, etc.)
(Fig. 11-1).

Ventricular septal defects produce loud heart murmurs, which facilitate detection. Unfortunately, these murmurs frequently are not audible
at birth or at the newborn physical examination, because the high neo-

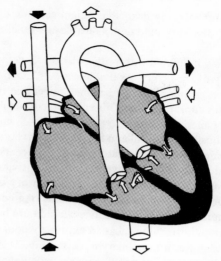

Fig. 11-1.—Typical ventricular septal defect high in the ventricular septum, allowing oxygenated blood to enter the right ventricle.

natal pulmonary resistance prevents much blood from passing through the defect. This hemodynamic characteristic always disturbs and confuses the parents.

Typically, the ventricular septal defect murmur is a grade-3 or grade-4, rough or harsh holosystolic murmur which is maximum at the fourth or fifth left interspace, next to the sternum. The murmur transmits well in all directions and is heard well over the back. There is frequently an accompanying thrill.

An infant with a ventricular septal defect, as an isolated lesion, may or may not have difficulty. The amount of left ventricular work in pumping the usual cardiac output plus the amount pumped through this leak in the ventricular septum depends on two factors: the size of the defect and the resistance to flow on the right side of the heart (pulmonary arteriolar resistance). The more blood flowing through the defect, the more immediate is the problem. Very large shunts lead to congestive failure, which is marked by poor feeding, respiratory distress, frequent lower respiratory tract infection, poor weight gain and increased perspiration. Moderate flows through ventricular septal defects may lead to slight dyspnea and a slightly decreased weight gain but do not usually lead to heart failure. Very mild defects may cause no clinical problems at all.

The chest x-ray in infants with ventricular septal defects will vary with the severity of the defect. As the defect gets larger or the abnormal flow becomes greater, the heart becomes larger and the pulmonary vascular markings appear heavier. This enlargement involves primarily the left ventricle and left atrium.

Treatment consists in careful and frequent observation and avoidance of respiratory infection. If a respiratory infection occurs, antibiotics (preferably penicillin) should be given—not to cure a viral infection but in the hope of preventing or curing a lower respiratory tract bacterial infection. If congestive failure ensues, it should be treated vigorously.

Cardiac catheterization during infancy should only be carried out if the infant develops heart failure, has an extremely poor weight gain or is suspected of significant pulmonary hypertension. The chief purpose of cardiac catheterization during infancy is to rule out an associated patent ductus arteriosus or a coarctation. These associated defects are found in 10% of cases. Either a coarctation or a patent ductus can be repaired early in infancy, thus removing some of the left ventricular work.

In rare circumstances, when heart failure is intractable or failure to thrive is severe, banding of the pulmonary artery should be attempted. This artificial increase in resistance to blood flow, if done adequately, will markedly reduce left ventricular work and lower the risk of heart failure.

Depending on the capabilities of the heart surgery team and the degree of pulmonary hypertension due to increased resistance, the usual isolated ventricular septal defect can be repaired after the baby reaches a weight of 20-30 pounds. The risk then is 2-5%.

A few infants with ventricular septal defects have or will develop very severe increased pulmonary resistance and will reverse their intracardiac shunt. Instead of the shunted blood going from the left to right ventricle, it will go from right to left ventricle. The child is then cyanotic and will show right ventricular hypertrophy; this condition is termed the Eisenmenger syndrome. Fortunately, this essentially inoperable condition only rarely develops in infancy, even in those with very large septal defects and very great pulmonary flows.

Patent Ductus Arteriosus

Hemodynamically, a patent ductus arteriosus is nearly identical with a ventricular septal defect. Both produce extra work for the left ventricle and left atrium, with cardiomegaly and increased pulmonary vasculature being proportional to the amount of blood going through the patent ductus from aorta to pulmonary artery.

The ductus arteriosus closes, as far as blood flow is concerned, in the first day or two of life in normal infants. In infants with respiratory problems or with hypoxia of any nature (e.g., from living at high altitudes) the ductus may remain open much longer.

In the older child with a patent ductus arteriosus one can usually easily detect the typical continuous (systolic and diastolic), or "machinery," murmur at the upper left sternal border or under the left clavicle. In young infants the murmur is most often a short grade-2 or grade-3 harsh systolic murmur that is loudest at the upper left sternal border but is also heard well under the left clavicle. Occasionally a short diastolic component can be heard as well. The pulmonic second sound will be normal to increased, depending on the pulmonary artery pressure.

Bounding pedal pulses indicate a patent ductus arteriosus of clinical significance in an infant. Normally an infant's pedal pulses are easily felt but are not prominent or bounding.

An infant with a patent ductus arteriosus will act the same as an infant with a ventricular septal defect, the clinical effect being dependent on the size of the shunt.

If a patent ductus arteriosus is suspected and is confirmed by cardiac catheterization, surgical correction can be offered if the defect is causing significant clinical difficulties. Even in small premature infants, a patent ductus arteriosus can be repaired at reasonably low risk.

Atrial Septal Defects

The common type of atrial septal defect (secundum type) rarely causes difficulty in infancy. The less common type, the so-called septum primum defect or endocardial cushion defect, may act like a large ventricular septal defect and lead to early difficulty. In the endocardial cushion defect there is absence of the lower part of the atrial septum, and there also may be ventricular septal defects and leaks or deformities of the mitral and tricuspid valves (called then a partial or complete AV canal). Although endocardial cushion defect can occur in any child, it is most commonly associated with the trisomy 21 condition (Down's syndrome, or mongolism). Approximately one in nine with Down's syndrome have this type of congenital cardiac defect.

Infants with endocardial cushion defect tend to behave like infants with large ventricular septal defects. Their murmurs are also similar, as are the chest x-rays. The chief help in suspecting an endocardial cushion defect is the electrocardiogram, which will almost always show left axis deviation plus right ventricular hypertrophy and a superior orientation (primarily an S wave in aVF).

This defect cannot be repaired or palliated in early infancy with any degree of success. After 2-3 years of age repair is possible in most cases, at a risk of 5-10%.

Obstructive Lesions

Less common, but still important in infancy, are the obstructive lesions. The left-to-right shunt group alone accounts for 40% of heart defects seen in infancy, and the obstructive defects account for 10-15%. The major obstructive lesions, in their order of importance in the neonatal age group, are coarctation of the aorta, pulmonary stenosis and aortic stenosis.

Coarctation of the aorta is the most common cause of congestive failure in the latter part of the first month of life. Conventionally, co-arctations of the aorta are divided into two types: the infantile, or pre-ductal, type, in which the constriction is above the patent ductus area; and the adult, or postductal, type. The "infantile" and "adult" distinctions reflect the tendency of the infantile type to cause more difficulty in infancy. The chief reason for the greater difficulty in infancy, how-ever, is the high percentage of cases of this type in which there are major associated cardiovascular defects. In the infantile type of coarctation, al-most all patients have an open patent ductus arteriosus and almost half have serious intracardiac defects (transposition of the great vessels, en-docardial cushion defects, large ventricular septal defects, single ventri-

cle). It is no wonder that a large number of those with preductal coarctations do not survive infancy.

Approximately half the patients with coarctation will get into difficulty early in infancy; two thirds of these will have the preductal type.
Respiratory distress and other signs of heart failure are the leading symptoms. Some 25% of the preductal group may have cyanosis.

Murmurs are not conspicuous in infancy. Half the infants have no
murmurs, and in the others the murmurs usually are not very loud and
frequently are maximum at the second and third left interspaces.

Although femoral pulses can be palpated in one fourth of infants with
coarctations, it is rare to be able to feel pedal pulses in the presence
of a clinically significant coarctation.

The blood pressure will be higher in the arms than in the legs, unless
severe failure is present. Unfortunately, reliable blood pressure readings in young infants are extremely difficult to obtain. Some of the
newer systems, using pulse detection or the Doppler principle, are
helpful.

As one would expect in the older child or the adult with a coarctation of the aorta, the electrocardiogram will usually show extra work by
the left ventricle (left ventricular hypertrophy). Most infants with symptomatic coarctations show right ventricular hypertrophy; this is especially true of those with the preductal type, because the right ventricle
is usually pumping against systemic resistance through a large patent
ductus arteriosus.

Infants with coarctation of the aorta who develop heart failure should
be treated vigorously. If there is no improvement in 24-48 hours of a
maximum medical regimen, catheterization studies should be carried
out and surgical remedy offered. If failure can be controlled or if the
infant is relatively asymptomatic, surgical repair should wait until the
child is 4-5 years of age.

Pulmonary Stenosis

Pulmonary stenosis is a not uncommon defect in association with
other cardiac anomalies, such as tetralogy of Fallot. When it occurs by
itself it is sometimes referred to as pulmonary stenosis with intact ventricular septum, or isolated pulmonary stenosis. If severe, it may lead

to reopening of the foramen ovale and allow blood to go from right atrium to left atrium, thus producing mild cyanosis.

Infants with isolated pulmonary stenosis usually look surprisingly well, even if the defect is severe. The marked failure-to-thrive appearance, characteristic of patients with large left-to-right shunts, is rarely seen in simple obstructive defects, even when they are severe.

A few infants with very severe pulmonary stenosis do develop congestive heart failure.

The murmur is almost always quite striking: a grade-4 or grade-5 rough ejection (crescendo-decrescendo) systolic murmur that is loudest at the upper left sternal border, with a thrill in the same location and in the suprasternal notch. The murmur is well transmitted. The pulmonic second sound may be difficult to detect because of the loudness of the murmur but is decreased or single.

The chest x-ray will show cardiomegaly if the stenosis is severe. On a lateral film this will be shown to be right ventricular hypertrophy. The main pulmonary artery, because of poststenotic dilatation, is enlarged. Pulmonary vasculature is usually normal.

The electrocardiogram is very helpful, especially in the severe case that is likely to be troublesome in early infancy. There will be a marked right axis deviation with tall, peaked P waves, indicative of right atrial hypertrophy in the precordial leads. In severe cases the R wave in V_{3R} and V_1 will usually be over 25 mm. in height. A strain pattern is indicated if deep T wave inversion is present through V_4 or more.

Heart failure, if it occurs, should be treated in the usual fashion. Although sudden death is rare, it can occur as the result of severe isolated pulmonary stenosis. For this reason a progressive strain pattern of severe right ventricular hypertrophy should call for consideration of surgical repair even in early infancy. Those patients with less severe stenosis can safely wait for surgical repair until they are 4-5 years of age.

Aortic Stenosis

Stenosis of the aortic valve, as an isolated defect, only rarely causes much difficulty in early infancy. A few infants with this defect will develop congestive failure.

The murmur of severe aortic stenosis in infancy can be misleading. Not infrequently, instead of being maximum at the upper right sternal border there is a grade-2 to grade-3 systolic murmur at the middle left sternal border—or even at the apex. Peripheral pulses, when the defect is severe, tend to be weak in all extremities.

The chest x-ray may or may not be helpful. Significant obstruction can exist with a normal-appearing heart.

The electrocardiogram may reveal left ventricular hypertrophy. Occasionally, in infants, right ventricular hypertrophy is also present. Significant stenosis can exist, however, with an apparently normal electrocardiogram.

Most infants with aortic stenosis do not develop severe problems in infancy. Those who appear to be severely afflicted should have a cardiac catheterization with pressure measurements across the obstruction. If the infant is in intractable failure or has very severe obstruction, surgical repair should be offered, even though surgical mortality is high. Those surviving surgery almost always have varying degrees of aortic insufficiency which probably will eventually require additional repair.

Cyanotic Group

Cyanotic congenital heart defects are those in which venous blood is somehow by-passing the lungs and entering directly into the systemic circuit: a so-called right-to-left shunt. As a group, cyanotic defects tend to be much more complex and more serious than the defects of the acyanotic group.

By definition, the arterial blood in cyanotic heart disease is less than fully saturated with oxygen (meaning the arterial blood has less than 92-94% saturation). This is not always the case, however: in such defects as truncus arteriosus there may be enough excessive pulmonary blood flow to keep the blood saturated.

Parents have great difficulty in detecting even moderate cyanosis and should be considered unreliable reporters when questioned about cyanosis.

After cyanosis has persisted for a while, clubbing (soft-tissue changes in the fingers and toes) develops. This usually takes several months and therefore, unfortunately, cannot serve as an early sign.

There can be other causes of cyanosis, of course, besides cyanotic congenital heart defects. For one thing, congestive heart failure from any cause, with its attendant slow circulation, can produce clinical cyanosis—usually a generalized dull-grayish color. The other common causes of cyanosis in early infancy are as follows:

1. Normal vasomotor instability, which can produce a secondary peripheral cyanosis or acrocyanosis.

2. Pulmonary causes, such as neonatal atelectasis, hyaline membrane disease, diaphragmatic hernia, lung agenesis, pneumonia and pneumothorax. If their condition is not too severe, infants with cyanosis secondary to pulmonary causes become pinker with crying or with breathing a high concentration of oxygen. In cyanotic heart defects, crying usually increases the right-to-left shunt and thereby increases cyanosis. Breathing a higher concentration of oxygen has little effect on the right-to-left shunt; therefore the cyanosis persists.

3. Neonatal neurologic problems, such as cerebral hemorrhage. This cyanosis is usually associated with irregular breathing patterns and other evidence of neurologic defects.

4. Methemoglobinemia, which produces cyanosis but no clinical distress. In methemoglobinemia the blood is a chocolate-brown color. The blue skin color will rapidly disappear if an oxidizing agent, such as methylene blue (1-2 mg./kg.) or 500 mg. of ascorbic acid, is given intravenously.

Clinical cyanosis is sometimes difficult to evaluate in the presence of severe neonatal polycythemia. With polycythemia there is a purplish, phlethoric appearance which becomes more pronounced with crying. If the baby is in any distress and the diagnosis of cyanotic congenital heart defect is being entertained, an arterial oxygen saturation should be obtained.

The cyanotic heart condition physicians are most familiar with is tetralogy of Fallot—the classical "blue baby" syndrome. The two chief defects here—severe obstruction at or below the pulmonary valve, hindering blood from getting to the lungs, plus a large ventricular septal defect—readily allow venous blood to shunt from right ventricle to left ventricle and aorta (Fig. 11-2). One fifth of infants with tetralogy of Fallot have complete absence of a pulmonary valve (pulmonary atresia). The pulmonary arteries themselves may have varying degrees of hypo-

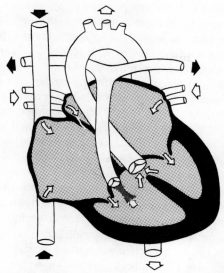

Fig. 11-2.—Diagram of typical tetralogy of Fallot with large ventricular septal defect, large overriding aorta and stenosis of the pulmonary valve.

plasia, which is a critical factor in surgery. Approximately one third of patients have a right aortic arch.

A few infants with tetralogy of Fallot get into difficulty with severe hypoxia, which causes dyspnea and easy fatigue. These are the infants with severe pulmonary stenosis or atresia. Occasionally heart failure occurs, but it is unusual.

Not commonly in the first month, but eventually, many infants with tetralogy of Fallot develop periods of intense cyanosis, hyperventilation and some disturbance of consciousness. These are variously called hypoxic spells, cyanotic spells or blue spells. It is extremely important that the physician recognize these episodes, because they can be fatal. The parents should be warned of the possibility and told what to be looking for. There is not a good correlation between the occurrence of these spells and the degree of cyanosis at rest: an infant may be intensely cyanotic at rest and never have spells, or he may be only slightly cyanotic at rest but have frequent spells. During these spells, either because of increasing stenosis in the pulmonary area or because of decreased peripheral resistance (allowing more blood to by-pass the lungs) the infant becomes progressively more hypoxic and then may faint, may have a seizure or a stroke, or may even die. In many, the eyes just roll up, and the infant is momentarily somewhat obtunded.

The physical examination in tetralogy of Fallot usually shows a fairly well or normally nourished infant with varying degrees of generalized cyanosis. Some with tetralogy of Fallot do not become cyanotic until they are more than 6 months of age. They may or may not be dyspneic at rest. They usually develop dyspnea after a little exertion.

Their heart murmurs may be due to the ventricular septal defect or the pulmonary stenosis, or both. Occasionally, with tetralogy of Fallot and pulmonary atresia, there are no murmurs.

The chest x-ray frequently, but not always, shows the wooden shoe, or coeur en sabot, configuration. This consists primarily of an uptilted apex of the heart (due to right ventricular hypertrophy) and an accentuation of the normal pulmonary artery concavity.

The chief thing to note on chest x-ray is the decrease in pulmonary vascular markings. The pulmonary artery markings tend to stop when about one-third or one-half the way out from the hilum. The right aortic arch, which is present in many, is strongly suggestive. If an indentation is seen on the right side of the barium column or the trachea, instead of the usual left-sided indentation, a right aortic arch is present.

The electrocardiogram in almost all cyanotic heart defects (except tricuspid atresia) shows varying degrees of right ventricular hypertrophy and right atrial hypertrophy. It is, therefore, not a great help. Normally, in tetralogy of Fallot there is a moderate right axis and moderate right ventricular hypertrophy. Right atrial hypertrophy may also be present. Left ventricular hypertrophy is not present.

What should one do with an infant suspected of the tetralogy who is doing well clinically (eating and growing fairly well and not having hypoxic spells)? If the diagnosis is fairly clear, it sometimes is safe to merely observe at frequent intervals. As a rule, however, the infant should probably have a cardiac catheterization and angiocardiogram, even if he is doing fairly well, to confirm the diagnosis and exactly determine the anatomy. The chief advantage of doing the catheterization studies early is to be able to proceed immediately to surgical operation if and when hypoxic spells occur.

The major indication for operation in infancy is to prevent further hypoxic spells. Once a definite or even a suspected hypoxic spell has occurred, the infant should be transferred immediately, with an "urgent" priority, to a center that has the team and facilities to operate on the infant heart. A shunt operation (either a Waterston or a Blalock) will probably be carried out.

If an infant does not develop hypoxic spells, the usual indication for this type of palliative procedure is to decrease cyanosis when it is severe and to increase exercise tolerance. Total correction of both the pulmonary stenosis and ventricular septal defect should wait until the child is 5 years of age or older. If pulmonary atresia is present, an aortic homograft can be inserted into the right ventricle and connected to the pulmonary arteries at the time of total correction.

If a child is seen during a hypoxic spell, he should immediately be given morphine sulfate (0.5-1 mg./5 kg.) plus oxygen. A knee-chest position may also help. In some cases morphine can also prevent hypoxic spells if given as soon as the infant becomes very irritable and restless, with increasing cyanosis.

If for some reason the palliative shunt operation is not possible immediately, the beta-adrenergic blocking agent, propranolol, may be tried. This can sometimes prevent further hypoxic spells. Beta-adrenergic blocking agents prevent the usual cardiovascular response to circulating catecholamines; therefore drugs of this class should be stopped 8-24 hours before general anesthesia. If the surgical operation must be done sooner, intravenous isoproterenol should be readily available to override this beta-adrenergic blockade.

Overcirculated-and-Cyanotic Group

Transposition of the great vessels is the most serious problem of the cyanotic congenital cardiac group of infancy. It is the most common cause of heart failure in early infancy and accounts for 20% of heart deaths in children. It is also the prototype of the cyanotic congenital cardiac defects that show over-circulated lung fields on x-ray.

In transposition of the great vessels (Fig. 11-3) the two circuits (systemic and pulmonary) are separate—not in tandem as they should be. The aorta lies anterior to the pulmonary artery, reversed from its usual

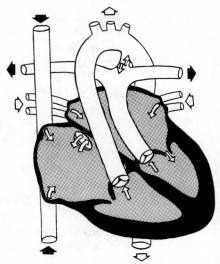

Fig. 11-3.—Diagram of transposition of the great vessels. The aorta arises from the right, or venous, ventricle; the pulmonary artery arises from the left, or · arterial, ventricle. An atrial septal defect is also shown.

position. This anterior aorta receives blood directly from the right (venous) ventricle. The left (arterial) ventricle receives oxygenated blood from the left atrium and immediately discharges this blood back into the pulmonary arteries.

This situation is, of course, incompatible with life unless a method exists for some oxygenated blood to get into the systemic circuit. This mixing of oxygenated blood occurs through defects of the atrial septum (in about 10% of cases, even though the foramen ovale is open in almost all), through a ventricular septal defect (in 25%) or through a patent ductus (in 50%). About one fifth of patients with transposition of the great vessels have such additional severe defects as single ventricle, tricuspid atresia and pulmonary stenosis.

Infants with transposition of the great vessels do poorly. Cyanosis is usually noted at birth or within the first few days of life and usually becomes progressively worse. Heart failure occurs in the majority within the first month. These infants have severe difficulty, with poor feeding, severe cyanosis, dyspnea and heart failure. Almost all die before 6 months of age unless corrective procedures are carried out.

The physical examination usually shows malnourishment, dyspnea and cyanosis. Murmurs, usually due to an associated ventricular septal defect or pulmonary stenosis, are prominent in only one third of patients. Another third have short, insignificant-sounding murmurs, and one third have no murmurs.

The chest x-ray is usually characteristic. The heart is greatly enlarged and looks like an egg lying on its side, with the smaller end toward the apex. The pedicle is narrow, and the pulmonary vascular markings are moderately or severely increased. All heart chambers are enlarged.

The electrocardiogram shows right axis deviation (except when associated tricuspid atresia is present). The P waves are frequently abnormal, indicating right or combined atrial hypertrophy. Right ventricular hypertrophy is present in the precordial leads in over half the cases—some of which have combined ventricular hypertrophy. During the first week or two of life the electrocardiogram may still be normal.

These infants require urgent cardiac catheterization to confirm the diagnosis and initiate treatment. The chief characteristic of an angiocardiogram is that the right ventricle discharges directly into the aorta, the left ventricle into the pulmonary artery. Lateral angiocardiogram shows that the aorta is anterior to the pulmonary artery.

Until a few years ago very little, if anything, could be done for infants with transposition of the great vessels. Now many can be saved by the following procedures:

At the time of cardiac catheterization a balloon catheter is placed in the left atrium through the foramen ovale. The balloon is then inflated and is rapidly jerked back into the right atrium. This procedure will frequently rupture the atrial septum and thus increase the intracardiac mixing of venous and arterial blood. When successful this Rashkind procedure increases arterial saturation about 10%. The risk is approximately 5%.

If the balloon-induced rupture is not successful or if the atrium gradually reseals in a few months, the surgeon can remove most of the atrial septum—another means of facilitating intracardiac mixing. This Blalock-Hanlon procedure carries a risk of 20-30%.

In general, everything possible is done to decrease hypoxia and control heart failure in these infants in order to get them old enough and
large enough for "complete repair." The procedures described above
(Rashkind and Blalock-Hanlon) do nothing to decrease heart failure.
Heart failure control must usually be medical, although in some instances
the surgeon can band the pulmonary arteries, thus decreasing left heart
work.

Total repair must be carried out before pulmonary hypertension becomes too severe. For that reason annual catheterization studies may
be necessary to determine pulmonary resistance.

Usually between the ages of 1½ and 4 years an attempt is made at
total repair. The procedure, devised by Mustard of Toronto, involves
placing a pericardial baffle in the atria to divert systemic venous blood
into the left ventricle via the mitral valve and, simultaneously, to divert
pulmonary venous blood via the tricuspid valve into the right ventricle.
Any associated defect, such as a ventricular septal defect or pulmonary
stenosis, is corrected during the same procedure. The mortality rate in
the Mustard procedure is still high, even in experienced hands; but
this may improve as the surgeons have more experience with this complex operation.

Hypoplastic Left Heart Syndrome

The hypoplastic left heart syndrome, even though rare among infantile heart defects as a whole, needs to be briefly reviewed, because it is
probably the most common cause of heart failure in the first week of
life. This condition consists of hypoplasia of various parts of the left
heart (as the name implies). This may include mitral or aortic atresia, a
hypoplastic left ventricle and ascending aorta. The left ventricle is
essentially nonfunctional; thus the entire heart load is carried by the
right ventricle. A wide-open patent ductus delivers blood to the aorta.

Heart failure usually occurs in the first few days. Cyanosis is mild
or moderate (rarely severe) and tends to occur later than the heart failure. More than half of the patients have no murmur, and the murmur
occurring in the others is not characteristic.

On x-ray the heart is seen to be moderately or severely enlarged, with
increased pulmonary vascular markings.

As one would expect with a nonfunctional left ventricle, the electro-cardiogram shows right ventricular hypertrophy, usually of a severe degree.

Even though the hypoplastic left heart is, at present, an inoperable defect, these infants should all have a cardiac catheterization with angiocardiogram to confirm the diagnosis. One always hopes that the clinical diagnosis will be found to be wrong and that something will be found which is operable. If the diagnosis is confirmed, the infant almost certainly will be dead by 2 weeks of age.

Congestive Heart Failure

Congestive failure is not uncommon in children. Most of the heart failure of childhood occurs in the first year of life, and 40% of cases of childhood heart failure occur in the first month of life. At some time or other approximately 20% of children with congenital heart defects will develop heart failure.

Certain heart defects tend to cause heart failure at different periods of infancy. The hypoplastic left heart syndrome is the cause of over 40% of failures in the first week of life. Transposition of the great vessels, co-arctation of the aorta, patent ductus arteriosus and pure pulmonary stenosis altogether account for another 40%. After the first week, coarctation of the aorta becomes the primary cause of heart failure for the rest of the first month. It is followed closely by transposition of the great vessels and endocardial fibroelastosis.

Infants with congestive heart failure show easy fatigue. When eating, they tire after one or two ounces of formula and must rest. They awake shortly and are hungry again. They are invariably irritable and usually restless. Their color is poor. In acyanotic congenital defects they may be a gray-ashen color or even slightly cyanotic.

Respiratory distress is always present. The depth of breathing is in-creased early, and retractions are common. Tachypnea, with respiratory rates up to 100, is usually present. In the late stages dependent pulmonary rales from heart failure may be present, but frequently the audible rales are due to concurrent infection rather than the failure.

The heart rate is rapid, except in congenital heart block or after treatment with digitalis. In the neonatal period heart rates usually go from

150 to 200 with failure. There may be a gallop rhythm—which is, however, difficult to hear at this heart rate. Heart murmurs are no help in diagnosing heart failure: the cardiac output may be so low that a previously heard murmur has decreased or disappeared.

The liver is enlarged. In the neonatal period a liver palpable 2-3 cm. below the right costal margin at the anterior axillary line is not uncommon. In failure the liver will usually be felt more than 3 cm. below this rib margin. The liver is firm, and on gentle compression the baby may stir as if uncomfortable.

All peripheral pulses usually are weak in the presence of heart failure. Peripheral edema or dependent edema is usually not detectable except when heart failure has long been present.

One of the problems in detecting heart failure in infancy is the inexperience of modern mothers in handling young infants. The rapid respiratory rate, which not infrequently will alarm the grandmother, is overlooked by the young mother. For that reason most pediatric cardiologists advocate the first well-baby checkup at 2 weeks of age rather than at 1 month of age. By 1 month, much of the heart failure has already occurred—and frequently is unnoticed until the baby is in critical condition (Fig. 11-4).

Except for the chest x-ray, laboratory data are not much help in diagnosing congestive heart failure. The chest x-ray, except in rare instances, shows some degree of cardiomegaly (usually moderate).

Although the electrocardiogram will not help to distinguish the presence or absence of heart failure, one should be obtained, inasmuch as it may give information regarding the underlying defect.

Hemoglobin determinations are useful, because a profound anemia can cause heart failure. A moderate anemia can certainly aggravate heart failure from any cause.

The treatment of heart failure in infancy is similar to the treatment of failure at any age. Digitalis is the mainstay of treatment; in pediatrics digoxin is the preferred form. For full-term infants I recommend a total digitalizing dose of 0.06-0.075 mg./kg., given in three or four divided doses intramuscularly over a period of 16-24 hours, depending on the child's status. Premature infants require only 0.05 mg./kg. Only very rarely is intravenous administration of digoxin warranted. Oral administration of digoxin is unsatisfactory in the beginning, because vomiting may occur, confusing dosage schedules.

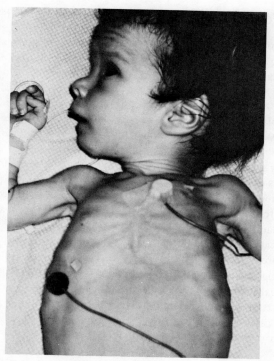

Fig. 11-4.—Infant in severe heart failure. Note the anxious look and the marked thinness, with lack of subcutaneous tissue and with intercostal and suprasternal retractism.

Babies being digitalized should be monitored in an intensive-care unit or at least should have a rhythm strip ECG before the last digitalizing dose, because arrhythmias signifying digitalis toxicity may occur. If an arrhythmia which may be due to digoxin is noted, the dosage should be cut.

If the baby is still in severe failure after a full digitalizing dose has been given and no arrhythmias have been seen on the ECG, a further one fourth of the digitalizing dose can be given every 12 hours until toxicity is noted or symptoms subside.

After the baby is fully digitalized, maintenance digoxin should be continued. The average maintenance dose is one third or one fourth of the digitalizing dose. This can be given in one daily dose; preferably however, a one-half dose is given twice daily.

If the infant is in severe heart failure or does not respond adequately to digoxin, a diuretic should be added to the treatment. In milder situations a trial of Mercuhydrin (0.1-0.2 ml.) or Diuril suspension (40 mg./kg.) can be tried. In more acute situations ethacrynic acid (Edecrin) (0.5-1 mg./kg., intravenously) has been found to be effective.

An auxiliary measure in treating heart failure in infancy is to facilitate rest by giving morphine sulfate (0.5-1 mg./5 kg.). Oxygen is helpful.

Feeding should be avoided in severely ill infants. They should receive fluids by vein but should not be given more than 2 mEq./kg. per day of sodium and potassium. After the baby improves, an experienced nurse can feed small amounts slowly. These infants fatigue easily and aspirate readily.

Pulmonary infection is, at autopsy, a frequent concurrent finding in heart failure of infancy. This justifies a therapeutic course of penicillin.

The prognosis of heart failure in infancy is grim: 50-85% die.

If the baby deteriorates or if he does not respond adequately within 24-48 hours of vigorous medical treatment, cardiac catheterization should be carried out, in the hope of finding a defect which is at least partially correctable.

LABORATORY FINDINGS

Electrocardiology

Although the electrocardiogram in the neonatal period is useful, it is not as beneficial to the diagnosis of cardiac enlargement as one would like. The many hemodynamic changes occurring in the first week or two of life lead to a large variation in the normal range of neonatal electrocardiograms. A single, apparently normal electrocardiogram in this period does not rule out significant organic heart disease. Serial electrocardiograms are more valuable.

Complete heart block is relatively rare. If the ventricular rate is over 50, then infants usually have no difficulty unless there is an associated underlying cardiac defect. Infants with ventricular rates under 50 may have either syncope or congestive failure. These symptomatic infants must be treated with a temporary venous pacemaker or a permanently implanted pacemaker.

The electrical axis in most normal neonates ranges from $+30°$ to $+150°$. An electrical axis outside this range would be grounds for suspicion.

The P wave should be less than 3 mm. in height. Tall P waves, 3 mm. or more in height, usually indicate right atrial enlargement. A broad, flat or notched P wave (over 0.08 sec.) is uncommon in early infancy but would suggest left atrial hypertrophy.

Most of the information regarding ventricular enlargement comes from inspection of the precordial leads (V_{3R} or V_1 to V_6 or V_7). The normal infant has predominantly right ventricular voltages; i.e., a dominant R wave in V_{3R} to V_1 and perhaps a fair-sized S wave in V_5 to V_6. There is a wide range of normal, but suspicion of right ventricular hypertrophy should be aroused if the R wave in V_{3R} to V_1 is over 15 mm. or if the S wave in V_6 is more than 10 mm., in the neonatal period.

Left ventricular hypertrophy should be suspected in neonates if there is a deeper S in V_{3R} than the R wave is high (R/S ratio less than 1), or if the R wave in V_6 is more than 16 mm. in height. A Q wave in V_6 of more than 3 mm. is also suggestive of left ventricular hypertrophy.

Evaluation of T waves can be particularly useful in the neonatal period. Normally the T waves are different in the first couple of days of life than they are the rest of childhood. The T waves are usually upright for the first day or two in the right precordial leads (V_{3R} to V_1) and then are inverted until teen age. Conversely, the T waves are frequently flat or inverted in V_5 to V_6 (left leads) in the first 24-48 hours but become upright after that.

Persistence of these peculiar T wave configurations after 48 hours of age usually indicates illness of some sort. It may mean hypertrophy of the underlying ventricle, or it may mean some chemical disturbance.

Chest X-Ray

Any infant suspected of a heart defect or disorder or who has respiratory distress should certainly have a chest x-ray immediately. Any infant with failure to thrive or evidence of easy fatigue (tires when eating) should also have a chest x-ray.

The most important problem with cardiac x-rays in infants is obtaining adequate inspiration. The infant's rapid respiratory rate, the inexperience with infants on the part of x-ray personnel, and occasionally the slowness of obsolete x-ray machines—these factors often leave us with chest x-rays in expiration or only partial inspiration.

One should always count ribs in reading cardiac x-rays. If the diaphragm is not down to the ninth rib, the film is essentially unreadable.

In reading cardiac x-rays we are, first of all, interested in the over-all heart size—the maximum transverse diameter of the heart compared with the maximum transverse diameter of the thoracic cage. In infants this should be less than a 1:2 ratio—if inspiration is adequate. Next, check the heart configuration.

The most important information to be gained from chest x-rays of infants with suspected heart disease is the relative amount of pulmonary vasculature (Figs. 11-5 and 11-6). Is it normal, decreased or increased?

Fig. 11-5.—X-ray of an infant with tetralogy of Fallot. Note the decreased pulmonary vasculature.

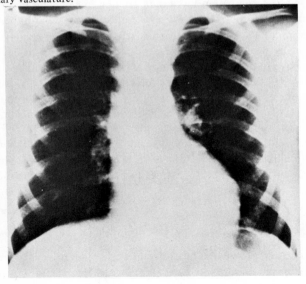

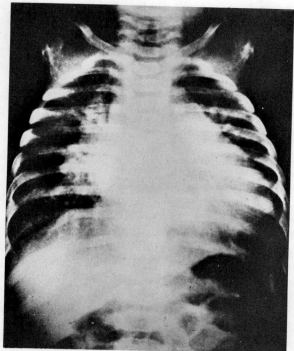

Fig. 11-6.—X-ray of an infant with a large ventricular septal defect. Note the large heart and the increased pulmonary vasculature.

Interpretation of pulmonary vasculature is difficult. A lightly penetrated x-ray makes pulmonary vasculature appear increased or heavy. An over-penetrated chest x-ray burns out or decreases pulmonary vasculature. And, of course, pulmonary infections, fibrosis, etc., can appear as increased pulmonary vasculature.

The best way to interpret pulmonary vasculature is to obtain a great deal of experience in looking at normal and abnormal infant chest x-rays. Even then it pays to be humble: we all make mistakes.

In the young infants, do not be satisfied with a single set of x-rays. The chest x-ray may appear normal at 2 or 5 days of age and yet show significant cardiomegaly a few days later.

How much can one tell about which part of the heart is enlarged when cardiomegaly exists? From the PA chest film alone, very little.

If the type of chamber enlargement needs to be known (and it does), take an electrocardiogram. Even though the ECG has its limitations as well, it is much more accurate for detecting chamber enlargement than an infant's chest x-ray.

Hemoglobin Determination

All infants in distress and all infants with suspected heart disease should have a hemoglobin assay, or hematocrit. A significantly low hemoglobin (8 Gm. or less) can lead to loud murmurs—either systolic or diastolic, or both. A very high hemoglobin (more than 20 Gm.) in the newborn period, with the associated plethora of polycythemia, may lead to confusion with cyanosis.

Any infant with congestive failure should certainly have a hemoglobin determination. Even a mild anemia (10 Gm.) in a non-cyanotic infant with failure can lead to more heart work. A careful transfusion of packed red cells (4-5 ml./kg. over a period of 2-4 hours may be helpful.

An infant with known cyanotic heart disease who has only 12-13 Gm. of hemoglobin has a relative anemia. Iron therapy (or, in exceptional circumstances, a packed red cell transfusion) may help greatly in decreasing failure or decreasing cyanotic "spells."

Blood Gas Measurements

Almost all hospital laboratories can now carry out blood gas studies on small amounts of blood. Arterial blood can be obtained from an umbilical artery catheter or from a radial artery. Arterialized capillary blood from a heel stick (warm the heel first with warm towels) may be adequate for determining the arterial oxygen saturation.

When one is in doubt as to whether or not the child has cyanotic heart disease, an arterial oxygen saturation can be extremely helpful. In the absence of hyaline membrane disease or some other cause of arterial unsaturation, an arterial saturation of less than 92% (19 vol%) would be compatible with cyanotic heart disease.

Acidosis can markedly decrease effective heart work. This deleterious effect of acidosis apparently occurs only in the presence of hypoxia. An arterial pH determination is, therefore, helpful in managing critically ill hypoxic infants. If the arterial pH is low, this should be corrected rapidly and rechecked frequently.

ADVANCED ASPECTS OF DIAGNOSIS AND TREATMENT

Consultation

One of the major decisions for the primary physician caring for newborn infants is when to request a consultation with a pediatric cardiologist. Because of the frequent need to carry out a cardiac catheterization on these sick infants, consultations should be requested from pediatric cardiologists with the training and the access to facilities and supporting personnel who can carry out cardiac catheterizations at any time of the day or night, any day of the week.

There can be no set rules about "when to refer" a child with heart disease. In general, however, any infant suspected of congenital heart disease who is cyanotic or has respiratory distress should be referred urgently to the nearest pediatric cardiologist. The younger the infant when the problem is recognized, the more urgent should be the referral: an infant who has already survived a month or two is less likely to deteriorate rapidly, but a 2-day-old may be dead in 24 hours unless urgent action is taken.

In spite of the proved ability of medical transportation to rapidly and effectively move combat casualties to the nearest medical center (so well demonstrated in the Vietnam war), we are still in the Dark Ages when it comes to moving sick infants. Perhaps the research now being carried out in the construction of specially equipped helicopters and ambulances for transporting critically sick infants will soon bear fruit.

Under the usual prevailing circumstances, a sick baby should be transported by the most rapid available means. During transportation the infant should be kept warm (monitoring temperature). If he is hypoxic, oxygen should be administered.

What about the young infant who is not clinically ill but who has a heart murmur detected on routine evaluation? Here again, there are no set answers. If the infant is not cyanotic, is not in respiratory distress, is eating well, has reliable parents and has a normal ECG and chest x-ray, careful observation should usually be adequate. If frequent observations of the infant, as well as his ECG and x-ray, show no difficulty, consultation can be delayed. Many heart murmurs of early infancy are transitory and eventually disappear.

Money should not be a consideration in determining the need for consultation in suspected congenital heart disease. Fortunately, all states have a Services for Crippled Children program under the auspices of the Children's Bureau; this program provides for consultation and for the care of children with heart disease whose families are medically indigent. The exact services and eligibility requirements vary to some extent in each state.

Cardiac Catheterization and Angiography

When should cardiac catheterization and angiographic studies be carried out on infants with known or suspected heart defects? The indications for such studies are much different in infancy than in childhood, when the risk is much less.

Primarily because of the critical nature of many heart defects in the young infant, the mortality rate for carrying out a cardiac catheterization in infants under 6 months of age is 5%, according to a recent broad study. After a year or two of age, cardiac catheterization, in competent hands, is a relatively innocuous affair, with a mortality risk of only 0.05% (1:2,000).

Because of the high risk in infants, these procedures should be carried out only in centers possessing a complete array of the necessary (and very expensive) equipment and staffed by experienced, board-certified or board-qualified pediatric cardiologists and heart surgeons. To decrease this high risk, it has been recommended by the American Heart Association and the Academy of Pediatrics that only centers performing at least 200 cardiac catheterizations on infants and children yearly, as well as at least 100 heart operations yearly, do these complex studies.

What are the indications for catheterization of infants?

I feel that any infant who is cyanotic because of suspected heart disease or any infant who has or has had definite congestive heart failure deserves a cardiac catheterization. The sicker the infant, the more he needs these studies. No infant is too ill for cardiac catheterization.

Everything possible should be done to get the infant into the best possible condition before doing a cardiac catheterization. These preparatory measures include correcting heart failure (if possible), correcting anemia and treating pneumonia. However, if the infant does not improve or gets worse in 24-48 hours, catheterization should not be further delayed.

If the infant has an obvious acyanotic heart defect but is doing relatively well (i.e., is eating and growing fairly well and has not been in failure), cardiac catheterization can be delayed until a time appropriate for possible corrective surgery. The ideal time for most elective heart surgery, I feel, is after 3-4 years of age. Not only is the risk less then, because of the child's larger size, but the psychic trauma of hospitalization is less.

Surgery

When should heart operations be carried out on young infants with congenital heart defects?

In my opinion, surgery in infancy should only be carried out when the surgical risk is less than the risk of medical management. No set answers can be given. Not only are the circumstances for each infant different, but the capabilities of each heart surgery team also differ.

In general, however, if the infant is in heart failure because of a large patent ductus arteriosus, he should have this repaired as soon as a trial of a maximum cardiotonic regimen has been carried out.

Infants with coarctation of the aorta who are in heart failure and whose heart failure cannot be brought under control within 24-48 hours of good medical treatment should also be considered for operation.

An operation which is feasible for the infant with acyanotic heart disease in early infancy is pulmonary artery banding. So far, repair of ventricular septal defects in the tiny infant, using extracorporeal circulation, has met with little success. Most infants with ventricular septal defects can be managed successfully medically. A few—those with intractable heart failure in spite of a maximum regimen—will be significantly benefited by the creation of artificial pulmonary stenosis (an umbilical tape around the main pulmonary artery). Unfortunately, this palliative procedure carries a mortality rate of at least 20-30% in this group of infants.

Even though the risk is high, an occasional infant with critically tight aortic stenosis or pulmonary stenosis requires operation in early infancy. If the infant is in severe failure and shows a strain pattern on his ECG, the risk of surgery (20-30%) may be less than the risk of relying on medical treatment. Such operation requires cardiopulmonary bypass and obviously should not be attempted by any but heart surgery teams with considerable experience in operating on young infants.

In essence, only two types of surgical procedures can be offered in the case of infants with cyanotic heart defects. The surgeon, with these tiny infants, can get more blood to the lungs for the hypoxic group with pulmonary undercirculation (as in tetralogy of Fallot). For those who are cyanotic with overcirculated lungs, the surgeon can produce better intracardiac mixing, thus reducing hypoxia.

Infants with cyanotic heart disease and undercirculated lungs are candidates for a shunt operation if and when they develop sufficient hypoxia to have "cyanotic spells." In very young infants the surgeon usually prefers to attempt a Waterston procedure, anastomosing the right pulmonary artery to the ascending aorta. A problem with this operation is that the surgeon may make the shunt too large, producing heart failure. In older or larger infants the surgeon can usually anastomize the subclavian artery to the pulmonary artery, thus increasing pulmonary blood flow and reducing hypoxia (Blalock procedure).

Infants with severe cyanotic heart disease whose lungs are over-circulated (as in transposition of the great vessels) cannot be helped by adding more blood to the lungs. To decrease hypoxia they need better mixing of arterial and venous blood in the heart. This can be achieved, at a risk of about 25%, by removing the atrial septum (Blalock-Hanlon procedure). This rapid procedure does not require extracorporeal circulation.

One hopes that within a few more years the heart surgeon will develop the ability to totally correct many heart defects in infants and not exceed the low mortality rate now achieved in older children. Most heart surgery in the older child can now be carried out at a risk of 2-5% for the noncyanotic group, and 5-20% for the cyanotic group.

Some heart defects, such as the hypoplastic left heart syndrome, can scarcely be remedied by surgical means. The only real hope in these cases appears to be an artificial heart or a heart transplant. Such procedures are probably at least 10 or 20 years in the future.

COMMON QUESTIONS FROM PARENTS

Cardiovascular disease, at any age, is associated with a great deal of anxiety. Parents and relatives of children with heart disease, therefore, have a great deal of understandable fear. They usually have a lot of questions which the physician should answer as best he can.

The following are questions I am commonly asked, together with my usual answers. Obviously, each child and each parent is different, and no pat answers are possible.

"How did this defect occur?" (What the parent is really asking is what did I or my husband or the doctor do wrong?) Parents should be told, whether they ask this question or not, that their child's heart forms between the third and ninth week of gestation; i.e., from the time the fetus is 0.3-2.5 cm. in length. During this time the heart changes from a simple straight tube to a four-chambered pump with two entering and two exiting tubes. It is no wonder that one in 140 have a defect at birth. The miracle is that the vast majority are normal.

The exact cause of heart defects is not known, in most instances. We do know that maternal rubella frequently leads to a patent ductus arteriosus or pulmonary stenosis. The trisomy conditions (Down's syndrome, trisomy E and trisomy D) usually have associated heart defects—frequently the endocardial cushion type or ventricular septal defects. Other chromosomal abnormalities, such as Turner's syndrome, also frequently have associated cardiovascular defects, including coarctation of the aorta and pulmonary stenosis.

The cause of 90-95% of heart defects is not known. Present evidence suggests that taking such common medications as aspirin, phenobarbital and antacids at the wrong hour of pregnancy may lead to various congenital defects. Certainly *all* drugs should be avoided, if possible, during the early part of pregnancy.

There is no evidence that anything the parents did, such as smoking or drinking, could have produced a congenital heart defect. They should be reassured in this respect.

The next question, which follows from the first, is: "Will this defect occur again in other children?" Luckily, there is very little chance that a heart defect will occur again in the same family. If one child has a heart defect, there is the likelihood that one other heart defect will occur if they have 50 more children! However, this risk of 2% for subsequent children rises precipitously if there are two with heart defects in the same family: the risk becomes 20%—one in five—that subsequent children will have a heart defect. Usually heart defects occurring in more than one child are of the same type.

Approximately the same risk applies to children born to parents who had a heart defect which was repaired. There is about a 3% chance that a child born to a parent with a congenital heart defect will also have a heart defect. Some defects, such as patent ductus arteriosus, atrial septal defect and idiopathic hypertrophic subaortic stenosis have a predisposition to run in families.

"Can my baby have baby shots?" In general, a child with a heart defect needs more protection—not less. He should receive the usual inoculations at the usual times, unless he has a cold or other infection. As with any infant, inoculations should be delayed if there is an infection.

"Can I let my baby cry?" Except in unusual circumstances, crying (or other physical activity) will not hurt a baby with congenital heart disease. If the baby has tetralogy of Fallot or other heart defect which tends to develop cyanotic spells, or if severe aortic stenosis exists, the baby probably should be "spoiled" and not allowed to cry for any prolonged period.

"Should I check him during the night?" Unless the baby has an obviously severe congenital heart defect, such as severe cyanosis or chronic congestive failure, the baby is not likely to get into difficulty within a few hours. "Crib death" or "sudden unexpected death" does not appear to occur in infants with heart defects any more commonly than in the usual child.

"What sort of food can we feed the baby?" Except in the very rare circumstances when we have to impose salt restrictions in infancy, babies with heart defects can and should eat the regular food appropriate to their age. In some infants there is easy fatigue with eating; in that case the baby might do better with smaller amounts of food at more frequent intervals.

"Can his brothers or sisters (or can we) play with the baby?" Again, unless the baby has an obviously serious congenital heart defect he should be treated as normally as possible. Unless someone has a fresh cold which he might give to the baby, there is no reason he should not be played with as much as is appropriate to his age.

"Can I travel with the baby?" Babies with significant cyanosis should not fly in airplanes or be taken to mountains. If airplane travel is necessary, oxygen should be readily available. Otherwise, unless the infant is in chronic heart failure there is no reason he cannot travel anywhere or by any method. If the baby is on digoxin, take an extra bottle or a spare prescription in case of breakage.

"Can I get life insurance on the baby?" I've been amazed by the number of parents who want to get life insurance on young babies. If the baby is thought to have a congenital heart defect, I know of no insurance company that would insure him. After a heart operation, if the defect is fully repaired, some insurance companies, but not all, probably would provide insurance.

"Will he be able to play football?" This question is usually from the father. If the child has a ventricular or atrial septal defect or patent ductus arteriosus, chances are that he will be able to take part in high school and perhaps college competitive sports, provided his operation has been successful. This is also true, but to a lesser extent, of those with pulmonary stenosis or coarctation. Children with aortic stenosis or one of the cyanotic heart defects are far less likely to have the stamina for such competitive sports even after surgery.

"What is the cost going to be?" An understandable cause for concern is how much the care and treatment of the heart defect might be. If and when cardiac catheterization is necessary, the family should figure on an average expenditure of about $1,000 (for hospital, doctors, etc.). If and when an open-heart procedure is necessary, the cost will probably be $3,000-$5,000 for everything. Closed-heart procedures, for patent ductus or coarctation, cost less. Nowadays, almost all reputable insurance policies cover these costs fairly well, even if the defect is congenital.

SUGGESTED READINGS

1. Cassels, D. E., and Ziegler, R. F.: *Electrocardiography in Infants and Children* (New York: Grune & Stratton, Inc., 1966).

2. Eliot, R. R., et al.: Heart Disease in the First Year of Life, in Cassels, D. E. (ed.): *Heart and Circulation in Newborn and Infants* (New York: Grune & Stratton, Inc., 1966), p. 243.

3. Glen, W. W. L., Browne, M., and Wittemore, R.: Circulatory Bypass of the Right Side of the Heart: Caval-Pulmonary Artery Shunt. Indications and Results, in Cassels, D. E. (ed.): *Heart and Circulation in Newborn and Infants* (New York: Grune & Stratton, Inc., 1966), p. 345.

4. Hallman, G. L., and Cooley, D. A.: Palliative Surgical Treatment of Complete Transposition of Great Vessels During First Six Months of Life, in Cassels, D. E. (ed.): *Heart and Circulation in Newborn and Infants* (New York: Grune & Stratton, Inc., 1966), p. 358.

5. Keith, J. D., Rowe, R. D., and Vlad, P.: *Heart Disease in Infancy and Childhood* (2nd ed.; New York: The Macmillan Co., 1967).

6. Krovetz, L. J., Gessner, I. H., and Schiebler, G. L.: *Handbook of Pediatric Cardiology* (New York: Harper & Row, Publishers, 1969).

7. Nadas, A. S.: *Pediatric Cardiology* (2d ed.: Philadelphia: W. B. Saunders Company, 1963).

8. Rudolph, A. S.: Biochemical and Hemodynamic Aspect of Cyanosis, in Cassels, D. E. (ed.): *Heart and Circulation in Newborn and Infants* (New York: Grune & Stratton, Inc., 1966), p. 173.

9. Smith, G. W., et al.: Banding of the Pulmonary Artery: Indications and Results, in Cassels, D. E. (ed.): *Heart and Circulation in Newborn and Infants* (New York: Grune & Stratton, Inc., 1966), p. 389.

CHAPTER 12

Metabolic Disease in the Neonate

HOBART WILTSE, M.D.

Inborn errors of metabolism have considerable importance to the physician who deals with newborn infants, but the low frequencies of these diseases tend to discourage systematic approaches to diagnosis. In three situations, however, an early diagnosis of inherited metabolic disease is both possible and desirable:

1. Phenylketonuria is a relatively common, treatable disease, and screening methods are available which are both efficient and economical. The success with phenylketonuria screening suggests that analogous technics should be in widespread use for such conditions as galactosemia and homocystinuria.

2. If an infant is born into a family in which an older child has an inherited metabolic disease, the physician will wish to resolve, as quickly as possible, the obvious question: does the apparently healthy newborn infant have the same disease?

3. Some inborn errors of metabolism are in a special category because of their ability to produce acute symptoms in the first few days of life. These are referred to as the "sepsis-mimicking" inborn errors, and the circumstances under which they deserve consideration are described here.

The chapter ends with a discussion of tetany caused by calcium or magnesium deficiency.

PHENYLKETONURIA: SCREENING AND DIFFERENTIAL DIAGNOSIS

The incidence of phenylketonuria (PKU) in the United States may be as high as 1:10,000 births. Diet therapy, if instituted early, can minimize or totally prevent brain damage. Diagnosis of all cases of classical PKU during the neonatal period is therefore a reasonable objective. All infants should be screened for PKU by means of a semiquantitative determination of the blood level of phenylalanine. Two test procedures currently available appear equally suitable: (1) the Guthrie test, a microbiologic inhibition assay in which the growth rate of *Bacillus subtilis* is dependent upon the amount of phenylalanine contained in a sample of the infant's blood; and (2) a fluorimetric assay of phenylalanine eluted from a filter-paper disk saturated with the infant's blood. Although the Guthrie test is older, the reliability of the fluorimetric method is well established. These tests are usually standardized so that a blood level of greater than 4 mg./100 ml. is reported as positive.

Ideally, the screening test should be performed after the infant has had 2 full days of formula feedings. Circumstances such as breast feeding, early dismissal from the nursery, use of antibiotics and poor feeding by some infants may leave the physician puzzled as to when a valid test can be best obtained. The screening test should *always* be done before the infant leaves the hospital, and any uncertainty about breast-fed infants or other infants who are dismissed before they are taking full feedings should be resolved by scheduling a repeat test at 3 weeks of age. Probably, most infants who will turn out to have classical phenylketonuria will have a positive screening test by 4 days of age, regardless of feeding history. Even with complete starvation, sufficient phenylalanine will usually be released by tissue breakdown to produce a significant elevation in blood phenylalanine. It likewise has not been shown that antibiotic therapy significantly interferes with the Guthrie test, and this should not be used as a reason for postponing the screening test. Performing a second screening test, routinely, on all infants at age 3 weeks is sometimes recommended but is difficult to justify in terms of likely yield of cases. A sounder approach is to aim for screening of all infants before they are dismissed from the hospital nursery, with repeat screening in selected cases at age 3 weeks to minimize the possibility of a falsely negative test resulting from a low dietary load of protein prior to the first test.

The time-honored procedure for testing urine with ferric chloride or with Phenistix has no place in the screening of newborns for phenylketonuria. The phenylalanine metabolites which appear in urine in an untreated case of PKU, namely phenylpyruvic acid, phenyllactic acid and phenylacetic acid, are not produced until an enzyme responsible for transamination of phenylalanine has made its appearance in liver tissue. Several weeks sometimes elapse before this enzyme becomes functional, and during this time an infant with classical PKU would remain unrecognized and untreated. Because the objective is early diagnosis and early treatment, no substitute has been found for a direct measurement of phenylalanine in the infant's blood during the first week of life. It is well to keep in mind, however, that the infant with classical PKU will have a normal blood level of phenylalanine at birth, because the placenta has efficiently maintained a normal level in utero. A screening test done on umbilical cord blood is worthless. The blood level of phenylalanine can be expected to rise slowly but steadily following birth and to rise quite dramatically once full feedings have been instituted, if the infant has classical PKU. Some laboratories have adopted the dubious practice of screening for PKU by means of amino acid chromatography of urine. Although this procedure might offer the advantage of screening for several diseases in addition to PKU, the probable benefit is too small to outweigh its uncertain reliability for early detection of PKU.

Considerable caution is needed in interpreting a positive result with the Guthrie test or the fluorimetric screening test. A positive result does not constitute a diagnosis of phenylketonuria, and further differentiation is required. Diet therapy with a phenylalanine-depletion diet is recommended for classical PKU and is often recommended for atypical PKU, but there are a number of benign conditions which produce a transient elevation in the blood phenylalanine in the newborn, for which treatment with a phenylalanine-depletion diet would be distinctly hazardous. The steps which are taken following the report of a positive screening test for PKU should, on the one hand, ensure a timely diagnosis and make it possible to prevent brain damage in an infant with authentic PKU, and should, on the other hand, avoid any possibility of brain damage resulting from inappropriate phenylalanine restriction in infants who do not have PKU.

The low-birthweight infant who receives a relatively high protein intake may have a transient elevation in blood phenylalanine—usually less than 10 mg./100 ml. but high enough to cause a positive result on the screening test. This can be caused by a temporary delay in the capacity to convert phenylalanine to tyrosine. More commonly it results from a temporary block in the pathway for further breakdown of tyrosine. Accumulation of tyrosine causes a secondary accumulation of phenylalanine; hence the positive screening test. Excess tyrosine in body fluids causes secondary metabolic pathways to come into use, beginning with transamination of tyrosine by the liver. The products of this reaction are chemical analogues of the metabolites which appear in the urine of the older phenylketonuric child. One of these tyrosine metabolites gives a positive reaction with ferric chloride or with Phenistix. This disturbance in tyrosine metabolism is known as "transient tyrosinemia," and during the first week of life *it is more likely to cause a positive ferric chloride test in urine than classic phenylketonuria.* This should underscore the warning given earlier: a positive Guthrie test is not diagnostic of PKU, and neither is the combination of a positive Guthrie test and a positive ferric chloride test on the urine. Rather, these findings are strongly indicative of the benign condition of transient tyrosinemia.

A further differentiation can be made by using a qualitative urinary test for phenolic compounds which are the breakdown products of tyrosine. In PKU, phenolic compounds are not found in urine because the metabolic block involves the conversion of phenylalanine to the phenol, tyrosine. Thus a positive test for urinary phenols (using a method such as the nitrosonaphthol test) is further proof that one is not dealing with PKU but rather the benign condition, transient tyrosinemia. The block in the tyrosine pathway occurs at a step which is dependent upon the presence of vitamin C, and administering 50-100 mg. of vitamin C daily to the infant usually causes the metabolic abnormality to vanish. Therefore, when the patient is a low-birthweight infant (or, occasionally, full-term), and the report is a weakly positive screening test for PKU, a very satisfactory approach would be to perform the ferric chloride test and the nitrosonaphthol test on urine and, if these are both positive, to prescribe the recommended vitamin C supplement and repeat the screening test several days later. Rarely, infants have been described who do not respond to the vitamin C therapy and are found to have a persisting abnormality in tyrosine metabolism. This is hereditary tyrosinemia, for which is recommended a special diet which limits intake of both phenylalanine and tyrosine.

If the steps described above do not establish transient tyrosinemia as the cause of the positive screening test for phenylketonuria, a measurement of the phenylalanine-tyrosine ratio becomes very useful. Normally, phenylalanine and tyrosine are present in about equal proportions in body fluids; i.e., in a normal ratio of 1:1. In classical PKU, where the conversion of phenylalanine to tyrosine is totally blocked, one finds a marked elevation in the ratio of phenylalanine to tyrosine. If the block is in the tyrosine pathway, the levels of both phenylalanine and tyrosine will be increased—but tyrosine more than phenylalanine, so that the phenylalanine-tyrosine ratio becomes significantly less than 1:1. Thus, when the screening test for PKU is positive and when the urine tests give no evidence to support a diagnosis of transient tyrosinemia, when the phenylalanine-tyrosine ratio is significantly greater than 1:1 and when the serum phenylalanine is significantly elevated by the specific fluorimetric quantitative determination, one has sufficient evidence to support a diagnosis of hyperphenylalaninemia, and a strong suspicion of phenylketonuria, either classic or atypical.

Further differentiation may not be possible until the infant is several months older, and it may be necessary to institute dietary treatment with only a presumptive diagnosis of PKU. The infant with classic PKU usually has a blood phenylalanine level exceeding 20 mg./100 ml. after a week or more of formula feedings, and the level will often reach 50 mg./100 ml. When this is the case, classic PKU is very likely. If the phenylalanine level remains below 15 mg./100 ml., however, one would more strongly suspect atypical PKU. In either instance, a phenylalanine-restricted diet is indicated to keep the serum level of phenylalanine below 8 mg./100 ml.; the diet should be instituted as soon as it becomes clear that it will be needed for this reason. Serum phenylalanine determinations should be done at semiweekly intervals for the first 2-3 weeks after institution of the diet, to prevent depletion of phenylalanine to levels below 2 mg./100 ml. When the blood levels fall to within the desired range, dietary phenylalanine in the form of evaporated milk is added to the infant's formula to provide 50 mg. or more per day of phenylalanine as needed to maintain the blood level above the lower limits. When a stable blood level is achieved, weekly determinations of the serum phenylalanine level may be sufficient until the infant reaches age 3-4 months. At that time, further diagnostic procedures are needed to exclude the possibility that the infant may have had transient hyperphenylalaninemia rather than PKU. Thus, a final diagnosis of PKU is not ordinarily made until an infant is several months old, but good management requires that the diet be instituted long before that time. If due care is taken in making the presumptive diagnosis of PKU, it is unlikely that any infants will be given a phenylalanine-depletion diet when they have no need for it and could be seriously harmed by it.

OTHER POSSIBILITIES IN SCREENING

Successful screening programs for phenylketonuria have generated interest in extending the screening of newborn populations to include other inborn diseases. Galactosemia screening, for example, appears to be technically feasible by the use of a procedure analogous to the Guthrie test for PKU. With little added effort newborn populations could be screened for both diseases, and similar technics have been devised for a growing list of inherited diseases. Plans for expanding screening programs to achieve coverage of several diseases should be based upon considerations of treatability, incidence, efficiency of the available screening technics and cost; in addition, the plans should take into account any effect the broader screening could have upon the success of screening for PKU. Depending upon the approach, broader screening programs might enhance the efficiency of PKU detection or might seriously compromise it.

Galactosemia

Galactosemia, with an estimated incidence of 1:30,000 births, is often nominated as the next most likely disorder deserving of routine screening in the healthy newborn population. The availability of effective dietary treatment supports this idea. But because, as will be discussed later, this disease characteristically produces symptoms during the neonatal period, one should appreciate that the yield of positive diagnoses is likely to be considerably less than the 1:30,000 figure if a population of *healthy* neonates is screened. Thus, a selective screening program for galactosemia with emphasis upon symptomatic infants, and using a technic which is simple and immediately usable at the cribside, may prove to be more effective in the early detection of galactosemia than a mass screening program in which the results of testing would be delayed a week or more in reaching the physician.

Testing the urine for reducing sugars by Clinitest after 48 hours of formula feedings is a procedure which should very satisfactorily meet these objectives. The decision as to whether the screening test will be performed upon all newborns or upon selected newborns who exhibit symptoms of disease should be considered at the time standard practices for any hospital nursery are being drawn up.

If routine screening for galactosemia is carried out by the Clinitest on urine, as recommended here, it is well to remember the existence of a benign condition known as lactosuria, which will occasionally produce positive tests with this screening procedure and will require differentiation from galactosemia. In infants with this condition, small amounts of lactose are absorbed but are not broken down to the component monosaccharides; thus the absorbed lactose is excreted in urine. All infants with a positive Clinitest should be placed on a formula which does not contain lactose or galactose, until the results of an erythrocyte assay for galactose-1-phosphate uridyl transferase are known. This test will confirm or exclude galactosemia. The galactose tolerance test is too hazardous to use for this purpose.

Homocystinuria

Homocystinuria is an inherited disease recognized more recently than either phenylketonuria or galactosemia. It is rarer than PKU but commoner than galactosemia. Untreated, it leads to mental retardation and other disabling complications. Dietary treatment may be beneficial if the intake of methionine is reduced. The enzymic defect involves a pathway in which vitamin B_6 is a cofactor, and in a significant number of cases of homocystinuria the administration of large amounts of vitamin B_6 corrects the metabolic defect. Although we cannot yet predict the outcome of dietary or vitamin B_6 therapy instituted during the neonatal period, the indications are sufficiently promising that any physician interested in screening newborn infants for metabolic diseases would do well to include this one. The qualitative cyanide-nitroprusside test on urine can be used, although its reliability in the neonate remains unproved. Two days of formula feedings should precede the test.

EXCLUDING INHERITED METABOLIC DISEASE

Because of low gene frequencies and recessive inheritance, the family history rarely provides help in the diagnosis of inborn errors of metabolism. The conspicuous exception to this generalization is when a sibling has a diagnosed ailment with known recessive inheritance. Under these circumstances the risk of recurrence is usually 25% in all children subsequently born to the same parents. This means that no metabolic disease is to be considered "rare" in a family already afflicted with it, and the question about whether a newborn infant has a disease previously diagnosed in one of his siblings can be an important question deserving a prompt answer. Under these circumstances early confirmation or exclusion of the diagnosis in the newborn infant is a reasonable objective, whether or not effective treatment is available for the condition.

In general, the physician faced with this problem is advised to bypass the common screening technics and proceed directly to more definitive diagnostic tests. For example, if an older sibling had a diagnosis of classic phenylketonuria, one would give the new infant 2 days of formula feedings and then obtain a blood sample for phenylalanine and tyrosine levels. Given a significant elevation in phenylalanine at that time and a significantly elevated phenylalanine-tyrosine ratio, one would have a presumptive diagnosis of PKU. If these metabolic abnormalities were not found, PKU would be excluded, and the parents would not be kept in suspense awaiting the results of the screening test and the stepwise procedures usually followed in the diagnosis of PKU.

Similarly, if an older sibling had galactosemia, good procedure with the new infant would involve avoiding galactose-containing formulas and making no attempt to screen for the condition by means of a urine test. Rather, a direct assay should be made for red cell galactose-1-phosphate uridyl transferase. In this way one would arrive at a diagnosis of galactosemia, or exclude it, without challenging the infant with galactose feedings. This appears quite desirable, because even small amounts may prove harmful to the galactosemic infant.

There are other times when available screening tests are simple to apply and when the more definitive diagnostic tests are so formidable that they are unlikely to be used at the time a diagnosis needs to be considered. Maple syrup urine disease (branched-chain ketoaciduria) is an example. Given a suspicion, based upon a previously involved sibling, that a newborn infant might have this condition, one might try to obtain an enzyme determination from a specialized laboratory soon after the infant is born and prior to the time feedings are started. Often, this will not be practical; so an alternative would be to cautiously institute feedings, observe the infant closely for symptoms of acute illness, test urine samples repeatedly for keto-acids by the 2,4-dinitrophenylhydrazine test and, if this test becomes positive, discontinue formula feedings and substitute glucose water until the diagnostic question is resolved with an amino acid analysis on serum to demonstrate elevation in the branched-chain amino acids. But if the feedings were well tolerated and if the urine test did not become positive, this screening test could be confidently used to exclude the possibility of maple syrup urine disease.

When parents have lost a child previously from one of the lysosomal (storage) diseases, they are likely to have serious anxieties about whether the new infant will turn out to have the same disease. Typically these diseases present no symptoms in the neonatal period; instead, there is a characteristic insidious onset and slow progression of the disease as the infant becomes older, leading to death in infancy or childhood, depending on the characteristics of the specific disease. Examples of these diseases include Hurler's disease, glycogen storage disease of the heart, Tay-Sachs disease, Gaucher's disease, Niemann-Pick disease, generalized gangliosidosis and metachromatic leukodystrophy. A feature of the diseases in this category is a general lack of straightforward chemical diagnostic tests. Also, the characteristic histologic changes are not likely to be present during the neonatal period, and attempts to arrive at a diagnosis by biopsy will usually be unrewarding. In most of these diseases, however, a direct enzymic diagnosis is possible on isolated leukocytes or cultured skin fibroblasts. When a storage disease is suspected in the neonate, these specialized procedures should be resorted to early, with the co-operation of an experienced laboratory.

Needless to say, a definitive diagnosis in the older sibling will simplify the process of investigating the neonate. The laboratory technics that confirmed the diagnosis in the sibling will usually be directly applicable to the infant.

THE SEPSIS-MIMICKING INBORN ERRORS

The transition from placental nutrition to oral feedings marks a time when some genetically determined metabolic diseases manifest themselves most acutely. The symptoms are usually nonspecific; i.e., they are similar to the symptoms that the infant uses to signal the presence of other kinds of illnesses, particularly infectious ones. The appearance of anorexia and vomiting, lethargy, coma, seizures, dyspnea and jaundice in any combination in the first few days of life usually suggests the possibility that the infant has septicemia. An unknown number of cases of metabolic disease masquerade as infection, and we must suspect that some deaths in the neonatal period attributed to septicemia are actually the result of an acute metabolic disturbance. Therefore, when clinical symptoms suggest septicemia, it is good medical practice to consider the possibility of metabolic disease as well. Because of the high early mortality in these conditions, rare diagnosis is probably not synonymous with rare disease.

The following is a list of some of the diseases which have been observed to produce fulminating illness during the neonatal period:

Galactosemia

Hereditary fructose intolerance

Hyperammonemia

Argininosuccinicaciduria

Maple syrup urine disease
(branched-chain ketoaciduria)

Hypervalinemia

Isovaleric acidemia

Propionic acidemia

Methylmalonic acidemia

Ketotic hyperglycinemia
(possibly synonymous with
propionic or methylmalonic
acidemia or both)

Some of these conditions produce a distinctive odor, and a deep sniff of the infant, crib or Isolette and diaper may provide an important diagnostic clue. Metabolic acidosis is a feature of many of these disorders. The physician who suspects a metabolic disease in an infant who has the symptoms of septicemia may find it helpful to have determinations made of the blood sugar, pH, CO_2 content and blood ammonia. Inexpensive qualitative tests on the urine, including the Clinitest, ferric chloride test and the 2,4-dinitrophenylhydrazine test, can be used to help exclude the possibility of metabolic disease when septicemia is being considered in an infant. It is useful to add to this a thin-layer chromatographic method for qualitative analysis of the urinary amino acids.

If any of the screening tests recommended above give positive results, it is wise to withhold further formula feedings, possibly temporizing for a day or two with glucose-water feedings or glucose by infusion, and seek further diagnostic assistance from a specialized laboratory.

TETANY

The signs of neonatal tetany include irritability, twitching, seizures and, often, laryngospasm. Carpopedal spasm and Chvostek's sign have little diagnostic value in the young infant, the first being frequently absent in infants with tetany and the second being demonstrable with significant frequency in normal infants. Of necessity, hypocalcemia (less than 4 mEq./L) or hypomagnesemia (less than 1.4 mEq./L) must be present; and unless the clinician has good reason to postulate a decreased level of ionized calcium in a "normocalcemic" infant, the diagnosis of tetany should always mean that at least one of these laboratory criteria has been met. Seizures of central origin usually have a more ominous prognosis than tetany, yet either may respond to intravenous calcium. An alert clinician will sometimes recognize symptoms of hypocalcemia (apnea, cyanosis) before frank tetany appears. More often, he will have to institute treatment for clinical tetany before he has established the fact of hypocalcemia. He should not permit this to hinder his search for causes.

Infants at risk—those of low-birthweight, those of diabetic mothers, and those whose delivery was complicated—are particularly subject to an early form of tetany which is not associated with a dietary phosphate load and may appear before feedings have been started. The basis is unknown. Classic neonatal tetany typically is several days later in appearing—always after feedings have been started and almost never affecting the breast-fed infant. Its relationship to the high phosphate content of cow's milk is well established, with some degree of transient hypoparathyroidism contributing to the susceptibility of some infants for developing this form of tetany. Maternal hyperparathyroidism should always be suspected as a possible, although unusual, underlying cause. Hyperphosphatemia (more than 7 mg./100 ml.) is as essential to the diagnosis of this form of tetany as is hypocalcemia.

Hypomagnesemia, because of a close relationship between body magnesium and serum levels, is probably synonymous in most situations with magnesium depletion. It should be considered whenever tetany occurs with normocalcemia or persists despite intravenous administration of calcium. Factors should be looked for which could account for magnesium loss in the mother; e.g., hyperparathyroidism, hyperthyroidism, diabetes, gastroenteritis and diuretic therapy. A few infants have been described as having a persistent, and apparently primary, form of hypomagnesemia.

Congenital diseases of the kidney sometimes signal their presence by the hypocalcemia which results from phosphate retention. Acidosis accompanying tetany should suggest this possibility, and the blood urea should be measured whenever this suspicion arises.

Treatment of frank tetany is by slow intravenous injection of 10% calcium gluconate (1-2 ml./kg.) at a rate not exceeding 1 ml. per minute, and always with continuous, direct monitoring of the heart rate, preferably by electrocardiogram. This dose can be repeated two or three times during a 24-hour period if needed to control seizures. Calcium salts are then added to oral feedings or are given by gastric tube, 3 Gm. per day in three or more divided doses, as calcium chloride, lactate or gluconate. Calcium chloride (diluted to 5% or less) offers the advantage of ready absorbability, but this may be outweighed by its irritant properties and the necessity to limit its use to 1 or 2 days because it produces systemic acidosis. Using correspondingly larger doses of calcium lactate will compensate for its poorer absorption and avoid the irritant effect of calcium chloride. The infant should be placed on a formula with low phosphate content.

Tetany which responds poorly to intravenous calcium or which occurs with normocalcemia and in the absence of alkalosis should suggest the possibility of hypomagnesemia. If confirmed by a low serum magnesium level, the condition can be treated by administering 50% magnesium sulfate solution intramuscularly, in a dosage of 0.5-1 ml./kg. per 24 hours, in four to six divided doses. The infant should be observed for possible hypotension following the injections.

Although the above measures will usually suffice, vitamin D in a dosage of 10,000 units per day is sometimes useful if tetany persists.

The use of vitamin D should be limited to 1 to 2 weeks' duration. If hypocalcemia recurs after vitamin D is withdrawn, this should alert the physician to the possibility of congenital hypoparathyroidism, and appropriate investigations should be undertaken.

SUGGESTED READINGS

Metabolic Problems

1. Berman, J. L., Cunningham, G. C., Day, R. W., Ford, R., and Hsia, D. Y-Y.: Causes for high phenylalanine with normal tyrosine in newborn screening programs, Am. J. Dis. Child. 117:54, 1969.
2. Berry, H. K., Leonard, C., Peters, H., Granger, M., and Chumekamrai, N.: Detection of metabolic disorders: Chromatographic procedures and interpretation of results, Clin. Chem. 14:1033, 1968.
3. Bickel, H.: Recent advances in the early detection and treatment of inborn errors with brain damage, Neuropaediatrie 1:1,1969.
4. Freeman, J. M., Nicholson, F. J., Schimke, R. T., Rowland, L. P., and Carter, S.: Congenital hyperammonemia. Association with hyperglycinemia and decreased levels of carbamyl phosphate synthetase, Arch. Neurol. 23:430, 1970.
5. Komrower, G. M.: Screening methods relating to inborn errors of metabolism, Mod. Trends Paediat. 3:85, 1970.
6. Menkes, J. H., and Eviatar, L.: Biochemical Methods in the Diagnosis of Neurological Disorders, in Plum, F. (ed.): Recent Advances in Neurology (Philadelphia: F. A. Davis Co., 1969).
7. Menkes, J. H., and Holtzman, N. A.: Neonatal hyperphenylalaninemia: a differential diagnosis, Neuropaediatrie 1:434, 1970.
8. O'Brien, D.: Biochemical Screening and Diagnostic Procedures in Mental Retardation, in Fried, R. (ed.): Methods of Neurochemistry, Vol. 1 (New York: Marcel Dekker, Inc., 1971).
9. O'Brien, D., and Goodman, S. I.: The critically ill child: Acute metabolic disease in infancy and early childhood, Pediatrics 46:620, 1970.
10. Scriver, C. R.: Diagnosis and treatment: Interpreting the positive screening test in the newborn infant, Pediatrics 39:764, 1967.
11. Shih, V. E., Levy, H. L., Karolkewicz, V., Houghton, S., Efron, M. E., Isselbacher, K. J., Beutler, E., and MacCready, R. A.: Galactosemia screening of newborns in Massachusetts, New England J. Med. 284:753, 1971.
12. Spaeth, G. L., and Barber, G. W.: Prevalence of homocystinuria among the mentally retarded: Evaluation of a specific screening test, Pediatrics 40:586, 1967.

13. Stanbury, J. B., Wyngaarden, J. B., and Fredrickson, D. B.: *The Metabolic Basis of Inherited Disease* (3rd ed.; New York: McGraw-Hill Book Co., 1972).

Tetany

1. Davis, J. A., Harvey, D. R., and Yu, J. S.: Neonatal fits associated with hypomagnesaemia, Arch. Dis. Childhood 40:286, 1965.
2. Ertel, N. H., Reiss, J. S., and Spergel, G.: Hypomagnesemia in neonatal tetany associated with maternal hyperparathyroidism, New England J. Med. 280:260, 1969.
3. Gardner, L. I., MacLachlan, E. A., Pick, W., Terry, M. L., and Butler, A. M.: Etiologic factors in tetany of newly born infants, Pediatrics 5:228, 1950.
4. Mizrahi, A., London, R. D., and Gribetz, D.: Neonatal hypocalcemia—its causes and treatment, New England J. Med. 278:1163, 1968.
5. Paunier, L., Radde, I. C., Kooh, S. W., Conen, P. E., and Fraser, F.: Primary hypomagnesemia with secondary hypocalcemia in an infant, Pediatrics 41:385, 1968.

CHAPTER 13

Transporting the Sick Infant

GEORGE BAKER, M.D.
G. VAN LEEUWEN, M.D.

The best-designed, most sophisticated, most reliable transport unit
is the uterus. One day, we hope, all pregnant women who are considered
at risk will be transferred, near the termination of their pregnancy, to
perinatal centers provided with modern equipment and well-trained
perinatal-health-care professionals. But even if that should come
to pass, there still would be a significant number of infants who, although their mothers had an uneventful pregnancy, would become ill
shortly after birth.

We must plan for the future but act in the present; and at present
we must contend with moving the sick newborn. This is quite unlike
moving the sick adult. Equipment, types of illness and required skills of
accompanying personnel are all different.

Most babies will be transported primarily by ground vehicles. For
distances of more than 100 miles air transportation is preferred, weather
permitting. We will deal primarily with equipping and staffing the
ground unit.

DESCRIPTION OF UNIT

One infant-transport van, developed at the University of Iowa Medical Center, is a modified van (International Harvester) which contains a
nursery measuring 6 feet x 10 feet x 6½ feet (Figs. 13-1 and 13-2). The
nursery-section walls have 2 inches of insulation, and an ambient temperature of 25-28°C. can be maintained by supplementary air-condition-
ing and heating units. There are two incubators: an intensive-care incubator (Air Shields C-86) with servocontrol and a transport incubator
(Oxygenaire). The intensive-care incubator is mounted permanently,

221

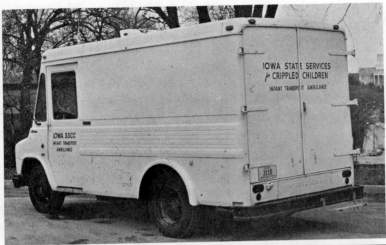

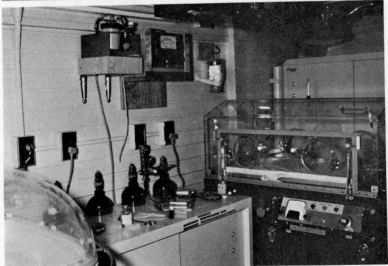

Fig. 13-1 (top).—Infant-transport van in use in Iowa.
Fig. 13-2 (bottom).—Interior of the van shown in Figure 13-1.

**Table 13-1. SUPPLIES THAT SHOULD BE ABOARD
AN INFANT-TRANSPORT VEHICLE**

Equipment
  Umbilical vessel catheterization tray
  Endotracheal tubes
  Laryngoscope with several blade sizes, extra bulb, extra batteries
  Hope resuscitator (or similar equipment) with several mask sizes
  Stethoscope (preferably one with electronic amplifier)
  No. 5 and no. 8 feeding catheters
  LP tray

Drugs
Ampicillin	Epinephrine
Kanamycin	Heparin
Sodium bicarbonate	Digoxin
	Mercuhydrin

Miscellaneous supplies
  Paper, for recording in transit
  Test tubes, for maternal and cord blood
  Parenteral fluids—$D_{10}W$, a hypotonic polyelectrolyte solution
  Needles and syringes
  Blood culture bottles
  Culture media

Information obtained at local hospital
  Maternal and infant records
  Identification bracelet
  X-ray films
  Laboratory reports
  Consent for operation
  Telephone numbers of referring doctor and the parents

but the transport incubator can easily be removed for transfer. Oxygen is provided in tanks, and suction is provided by a pump aspirator. Several battery-operated cardiotachometers have been used. A gasoline-powered generator is mounted under the floor; it is rated by the manufacturer at 10.4 amperes and 110 volts. A back-up system provides lighting from either the auxiliary generator, the van's electrical system or a battery-powered light. In case of failure of the main generator, lighting can be provided from the van's electrical system or by a battery-powered lamp. Suction can be managed by hand with a trap (DeLee), if necessary.

Resuscitation equipment, drugs and intravenous fluids are available in a central work space. Two-way radio communication, by way of the highway patrol, permits consultation or the alerting of the hospital as to special needs on arrival. Because speed is not a primary concern, patrol escort is not normally sought. The unit used at The University of Nebraska Medical Center is similar in design.

The initial cost of the van, its modification and its basic equipment was $12,600. Operational costs are in large part dependent on the use of personnel for other duties when the van is not in use. If the driver works in the hospital as an orderly when not operating the van, and if nursing and medical personnel are also employed at other duties, the cost is approximately 80 cents per mile, including depreciation of all equipment. If the driver is paid for on-call time exclusively, from the van operating account, cost per mile climbs to approximately $1.50.

In the absence of a specifically designed emergency transport van, many improvisations are possible. Provided a skilled person, the equipment listed in Table 13-1 and an infant-transport incubator are present, babies can be moved reasonably well in almost any vehicle: we have used station wagons, sedans, vans and even a Volkswagen.

OPERATION

The transport van we have been describing serves an area of 100-mile radius. Beyond this, transfer is probably best accomplished by air. A driver and a physician are on 24-hour call, to facilitate transfer at any time. A nurse may accompany the physician if problems requiring extra help are anticipated. For the transfer of infants from the medical center back to outlying hospitals for convalescent care, a nurse is in attendance alone.

Upon call from a referring physician, the van is dispatched soon—usually within 30 minutes. Most infants tolerate the 2-hour delay from time of referral until care can be instituted in the van.

A medical history and a report of medical management prior to transfer are obtained at the time of transfer. This information includes the maternal history (medications, pregnancy, labor and delivery status) as well as the history of infant's subsequent condition and course. Appropriate cultures and roentgenograms accompany the infant.

The physician who is to make the trip evaluates the infant in the nursery and then transfers him to the van. He may spend further time in evaluation, in clearing the airway or in initiating therapy before the van leaves the hospital. En route, if problems arise the van is slowed or stopped while the infant is cared for. Consultation with the center should be possible by radio, if necessary.

The transportation system described is designed to meet the medical needs of infants in a semirural region. It extends the special facilities and personnel of a medical center to the region in which it operates. The system permits medical evaluation and treatment to begin when the infant is admitted to the van. Infants who require admission to a medical center can receive constant attention by medical personnel en route. At times, diagnoses are made and therapy is started before arrival.

Because convalescence in the community hospital permits the family to participate in patient care, the van should be used to transfer the infants from the center to community hospitals where they can be under the care of the referring physician, as soon as they are sufficiently recovered.

Several problems have arisen during the development of the transport system. Road noise precludes auscultation of the heart; thus a cardiotachometer is necessary. Rough roads, especially in the winter, have resulted in a somewhat more bouncy ride than is desirable; so a belt of nylon was devised for the infant, to restrict his movement in the incubator. However, no identifiable medical problems have arisen as a result of a rough ride.

Laboratory equipment has not been used in the system. There is the problem of mounting such equipment; and besides, we have seldom needed laboratory work en route. Sodium bicarbonate has been given intravascularly, using an empirical dosage for infants in distress. Consideration is being given to the need for a blood gas analysis in the van.

As for other uses of such a transport system: (1) infants transported by air from more than 100 miles may be carried by van transfer from the airport to the hospitals; and (2) the system, although designed for a semirural region, is equally useful in a city or its suburbs.

AIR TRANSPORTATION

Transporting infants by air poses additional problems: lighting is less satisfactory, working space is limited, air travel is costly, and weather often interferes. Once perinatal centers are established so that infants are born near if not in the center, there will be even less need for air transportation. In large cities, helicopters may have a valuable role in hospital-to-hospital transfer, but because of cost and lack of adequate space they have minimal usefulness in less congested places.

Infants with certain conditions, notably pneumothorax and pneumomediastinum, are subject to special risk at high altitudes in unpressurized aircraft.

Except under unusual circumstances, we doubt whether the cost of purchasing, operating and staffing an air ambulance is justified. We have also found that when we need air transportation, many people offer their services. The Air Force, National Guard, police, private pilots, members of our faculty who are pilots—all volunteered their services when asked.

SUMMARY

We would like to stress the following points:

1. The transport unit should be based at the receiving center. This insures that the personnel and equipment will be appropriate to the infant's needs.

2. A physician or a nurse skilled in the care of newborns should accompany the baby. A fairly simple unit cannot be converted into an intensive-care unit with more equipment alone, but it can become one if a skilled professional is present. Only nurses who are trained in intubation and umbilical vessel catheterization should be considered sufficiently skilled to substitute for a physician.

3. We believe that some laboratory equipment, especially a centrifuge for hematocrit determination, should be on board. Equipment for analyzing blood gases is bulky, expensive and sensitive, but because of potential urban traffic congestion it may be necessary.

4. Air transport of sick infants has a limited future, except possibly for helicopter transport in large cities.

5. With a suitable vehicle, such as the one described here, and a skilled physician or nurse in attendance, much of the stress involved in transporting the sick infant can be relieved. Speed of transit becomes progressively less important as the unit becomes refined so that intensive care can be delivered in transit.

SUGGESTED READINGS

1. Segal, S.: Transfer of a premature or other high risk newborn infant to a referral hospital, Pediat. Clin. North America 13:1195, 1966.
2. Baker, G. L.: Design and operation of a van for the transport of sick infants, Am. J. Dis. Child. 118:743, 1969.

CHAPTER 14

Procedures

G. VAN LEEUWEN, M.D.

This chapter briefly describes the procedures frequently used in newborn infants for diagnosis and therapy, with appropriate illustrations.
The procedures described are lumbar puncture, umbilical vessel catheterization, femoral vein puncture, external and internal jugular puncture,
scalp vein entry, radial artery puncture, suprapubic bladder aspiration,
thoracentesis, lung puncture and subdural puncture.

LUMBAR PUNCTURE

The technic of obtaining cerebrospinal fluid from the small infant
atraumatically is difficult and cannot be mastered without doing the
procedure repeatedly. Our technic is to put the infant in a sitting position and to enter one interspace above the level of the iliac crest
(Fig. 14-1). The subarachnoid space which contains fluids is larger
proximally than at the iliac crest. The area is prepared in the usual
manner; then a 22-gauge needle with stylet is inserted through the skin.
Immediately after perforating the skin, the stylet is removed and the
needle is advanced almost at right angles to the infant (not in a
cephalad direction, as in adults). The needle should be advanced so
slowly that an observer would not notice that it is moving. There is
usually no feeling of entering the subarachnoid space, by comparison
with the slight sense of puncturing the membrane in older patients. For
this reason, with each millimeter of advancement the needle is rotated
and the operator waits 5-10 seconds before advancing farther. In this
way nonbloody spinal fluid can be obtained. We usually remove a very
small amount: just enough for cell count, culture, and protein and glucose determination. This can be done as part of the culturing process

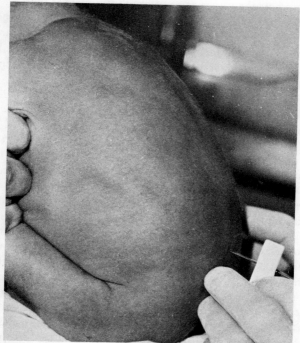

Fig. 14-1.—The most satisfactory position for lumbar puncture. With the infant sitting up, the needle is more easily kept in the midline. The entering point for lumbar puncture is one or two interspaces above the iliac crest. Many prefer entering lower, but we have had best results in this area.

for septicemia. If only a few drops of fluid can be obtained, this is examined for organisms and sent for culture. Using a scalp vein needle is also a satisfactory method.

UMBILICAL ARTERY AND VEIN PROCEDURES

The umbilical vein is still used to perform exchange transfusions. Entering the vein is a simple procedure, best done after the cord has been cut almost flush with the abdomen (Fig. 14-2). A no. 5 or no. 8 radiopaque catheter is used. For exchange transfusions one tries to go only as far as is necessary to obtain easy withdrawal of blood. In other situations, where the vein is being utilized to administer fluid, the catheter is very carefully advanced through the liver via the ductus venosus into the inferior vena cava or right atrium. This position is ascertained by x-ray prior to the instillation of solutions other than glucose. Hypertonic solutions given directly into the liver result in necrosis of the liver in animals and presumably are not safe to give to humans.

Catheterization of the umbilical artery is considerably more difficult and should never be attempted by an inexperienced physician. Our technic is to expose the artery, grasp each wall with a very small hemostat or arterial clamp, and then drop iris scissors into the lumen to dilate the lumen sufficiently to permit entrance of the catheter. After this dilatation is accomplished, a no. 5 or no. 3½ radiopaque umbilical catheter is inserted (Fig. 14-3). The only point of obstruction is usually at the junction of the iliac and umbilical arteries. Firm rotational pressure (do not use a metal probe) will usually break this spasm and permit the turn to be made. The catheter is then advanced until it is opposite the tenth thoracic vertebra, in the thoracic aorta. Again x-rays are made and the position of the catheter is ascertained before hypertonic solutions are administered.

The umbilical vein catheter should not be left in place more than 72 hours, because of the likelihood of infection. The arterial catheter appears less likely to become infected and can be left in for several days. It should, however, be removed as soon as blood gas determinations are no longer needed.

When the catheter is removed, firm pressure for 2-3 minutes will control any hemorrhage from either the vein or the artery; suturing is not usually necessary. We do not routinely administer antibiotics during or after either umbilical vein or arterial catheterization.

FEMORAL VEIN PUNCTURE

Because of the danger to the joint space and the reported incidence of arteriovenous fistula, we rarely use the femoral vein or artery for diagnostic procedures. When we do, we use a 21-gauge scalp needle to puncture the vein. The capillary action in the plastic tubing permits blood to come forth immediately when the vessel is entered; this minimizes the amount of trauma which takes place. This technic is illus-

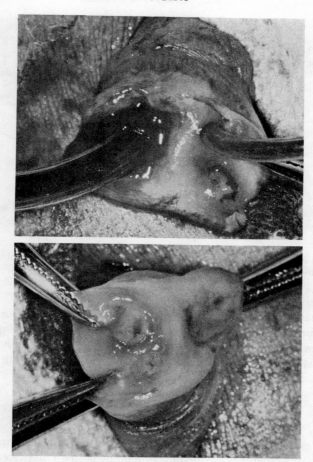

Fig. 14-2 (top).—Closeup of the umbilical stump, showing the anatomic relationship of the two arteries opposite the large vein.

Fig. 14-3 (bottom).—Closeup of umbilical stump, showing a no. 8 catheter in the vein and a no. 5 catheter in the artery.

trated in Figure 14-4. When femoral artery puncture for blood gas determination is attempted, the same procedure is used, except that the needle is inserted slightly laterally. Again, we wish to emphasize that this procedure should rarely be done. It is done most easily if the in-

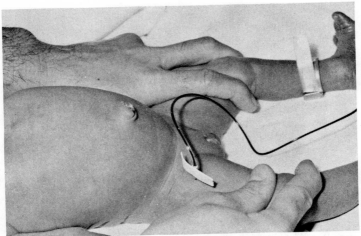

Fig. 14-4.—Technic of femoral vein puncture, using a 21-gauge scalp needle. This method is considerably less traumatic than other methods.

fant's legs are at a 45° angle to the trunk and are abducted to 90°. This is illustrated in the photograph. Firm pressure must be applied for several minutes after withdrawal of the needle, to prevent the development of a hematoma. Occasionally after arterial puncture the extremity becomes white secondary to arterial spasm. This can be treated with warm compresses, and response is usually prompt.

EXTERNAL JUGULAR PUNCTURE

The external jugular vein is readily accessible in the small infant and can be easily entered if the infant is held in the position illustrated in Figure 14-5. Both shoulders must be flat on a hard surface, with the head turned at right angles and slightly flexed while it is hanging over the edge of the hard surface. The skin should be entered about 1 cm. proximal to the desired point of entry into the vein; and then, while the infant is crying, deliberate stabbing at the vein is more successful than gentle entry. Up to 10 ml. of blood can usually be aspirated. On rare occasions blood or fluids may be administered by push through this vein.

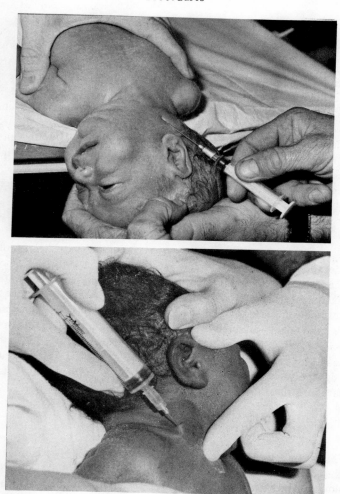

Fig. 14-5 (top).—Point of entry for external jugular puncture. Note that the shoulders are flat on the table. The same position is used for internal jugular puncture, but the point of entry is beneath and behind the sternocleidomastoid muscle.

Fig. 14-6 (bottom).—Demonstration of the midpoint of the internal jugular puncture, with the tip of the needle palpable in the suprasternal notch.

INTERNAL JUGULAR PUNCTURE

This procedure is rarely necessary, but it provides a ready access to large amounts of blood. The positioning is identical with that for external jugular puncture. A long 20-gauge needle is inserted through the skin behind and under the sternocleidomastoid muscle. The needle is advanced to the suprasternal notch, where it should be palpable just under the skin by the index finger (Fig. 14-6). As the syringe and needle are withdrawn, the internal jugular will be traversed. This procedure can be dangerous: occasionally the trachea is entered, and this may result in an immediate respiratory arrest requiring resuscitation. Again, we discourage the use of this procedure except under unusual circumstances.

SCALP VEIN PROCEDURES

Although scalp veins are difficult to locate in the first 24 hours of life, because of scalp edema, thereafter they are readily accessible both for the instillation of fluids and for the withdrawal of small amounts of blood. A rubber band is placed around the infant's head, just above the ears; this distends the veins and makes them readily visible. The arteries in the scalp are not affected by this procedure, and therefore the operator is less likely to enter one. A short, beveled no. 21 or no. 23 needle is used, and the vein is entered and threaded (Fig. 14-7). To prevent easy dislodging of the vein, a small plastic medicine cup or paper cup is taped in place over the area (Fig. 14-8).

RADIAL ARTERY PUNCTURE

This is a relatively new technic which, if developed, may eliminate much of the need for umbilical artery catheterization. Arterial oxygen tension measurements are probably more accurate from the radial artery particularly, if one is concerned about the amount of oxygen going to the brain. The right radial artery is used, because of the anatomic distribution of the great vessels. A short, beveled 25-gauge needle on a syringe is used, and the skin is entered immediately adjacent to the styloid process of the radius at an angle of about 45° (Fig. 14-9). The artery often goes into spasm; therefore, when one feels that the artery

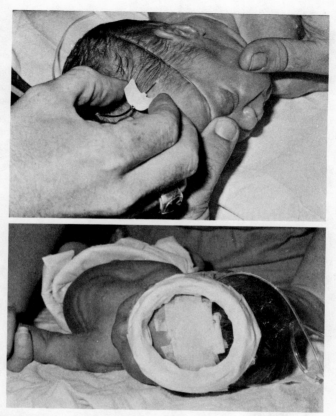

Fig. 14-7 (top).—Technic of entering a scalp vein. Note the rubber band, used as a tourniquet.

Fig. 14-8 (bottom).—One method of protecting a scalp vein infusion: using part of a paper cup.

has been entered one should wait for a moment before attempting another puncture, inasmuch as the needle may be in the lumen of the vessel. One to two milliliters of blood, sufficient for blood gas determinations, can be withdrawn from the radial artery. This procedure can be repeated at 4-hour intervals, apparently, without any permanent damage resulting to the radial artery.

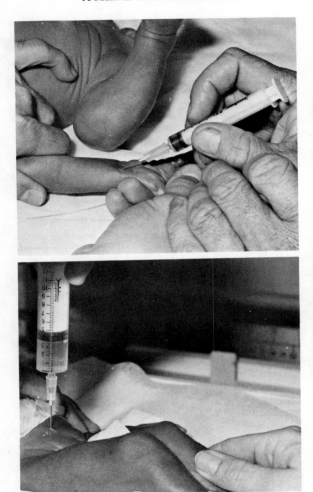

Fig. 14-9 (top).—Technic of entering the radial artery with a 23-gauge needle, adjacent to the styloid process, at a 45° angle.

Fig. 14-10 (bottom).—Suprapubic aspiration of urine. The needle is placed about 1 cm. above the symphysis pubis.

SUPRAPUBIC BLADDER ASPIRATION

This harmless procedure provides a quick means of obtaining urine for examination and culture. The abdomen is prepared as for a blood culture; i.e., with iodine and alcohol. A gloved index finger is placed on the upper portion of the pubic bone, and the needle is inserted about one fingerbreadth above the top of the pubis. The needle then should enter at right angles to the table (Fig. 14-10). If one goes straight down, the bladder neck is entered and no urine will be obtained.

A 21-gauge needle is used, and aspiration is accomplished both on entry and exit. An assistant should occlude the urethral opening from the beginning of preparation of the skin, simply because stimulation in this area usually results in micturition. One should also be certain that the infant has not wet his diaper during the hour before the procedure is attempted. Rarely, fecal material is obtained on aspiration, but this appears not to harm the infant; at least, we have not encountered any complications from this. One episode of microscopic hematuria is not uncommon following this procedure and should not be interpreted with alarm.

THORACENTESIS

Thoracentesis in the newborn infant is largely reserved for the baby with tension pneumothorax. We now perform this procedure with a no. 18 or no. 20 needle anteriorly in about the second intercostal space, with the infant in a sitting position (Fig. 14-11). A three-way stopcock must be used, so that the amount of air removed can be measured and discharged. Should the pneumothorax immediately recur and a second aspiration be necessary, we use an intracatheter as the chest tube, rather than one of the old-style large tubes. This has been completely satisfactory in keeping the pleural space empty of air and permitting expansion of the lung. If this procedure is done on a critically ill infant, one should pay careful attention to the arterial oxygen tension after the lung has expanded, because the tension may increase rapidly.

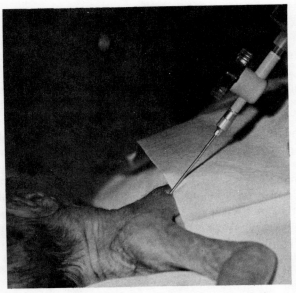

Fig. 14-11.—Apical thoracentesis technic used in treating tension pneumo-thorax.

LUNG PUNCTURE

Diagnostic lung puncture has become increasingly popular in recent years. We have not found this to be a very satisfactory procedure in the newborn, although we continue to perform it when we are not certain of the diagnosis. One should use a 20-gauge needle on a syringe containing about 0.5 ml. of saline. The side which one wants to puncture is approached, and aspiration is begun the moment the needle has penetrated the skin (Fig. 14-12). In about 5 seconds the needle is inserted and withdrawn. The needle and the saline in the syringe are then cultured.

We have not attempted lung biopsies by direct puncture in newborns, but we have used this method to obtain material for culturing. Our results have been very unsatisfactory in providing answers; however, the procedure itself does not seem to harm the infant or produce any pneumothorax. In all lung punctures the hole should be sealed after withdrawal of the needle, to prevent iatrogenic pneumothorax.

SUBDURAL PUNCTURE

Subdural puncture is one of the easier procedures in the newborn if proper equipment is used. The short needles designed for subdural taps are best. The scalp is shaved and prepared in the usual fashion; then the most lateral portion of the anterior fontanelle is located. The needle is inserted at the suture line or in the most lateral corner of the anterior fontanelle (Fig. 14-13). The characteristic pop is felt as the needle penetrates. A hemostat should then be clamped on, so that the needle is not inadvertently inserted farther. The needle is pointed anteriorly, laterally and posteriorly. Absence of fluid or the presence of 1-2 ml. of straw-colored fluid is considered normal. In the small, dehydrated infant who does not have subdural hemorrhage or subdural collection of fluid it is very easy to injure the cerebral cortex if one is not careful to stop immediately after the pop is felt.

Fig. 14-12.– Diagnostic lung puncture, using a 20-gauge needle. Aspiration is started as soon as the skin is perforated and is continued during the in-and-out maneuver.

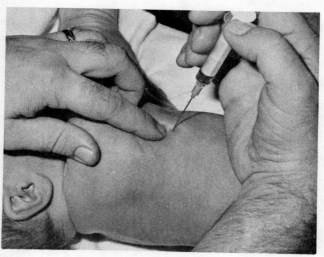

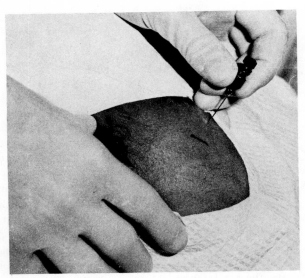

Fig. 14-13.—Subdural puncture. Note that the operator is inserting the needle as far laterally as possible.

Acknowledgment

The author wishes to express his thanks to Dr. Charles Elfont for doing much of the photography involved in developing this chapter.

CHAPTER 15

Total Intravascular Alimentation

G. VAN LEEUWEN, M.D.

Early feeding intravenously or intraarterially, using 10% glucose, has been shown to reduce the mortality rate in small premature infants. This is a form of total intravascular alimentation, but it is a very safe and relatively mild form. Because of the recent reports of parenteral alimentation sustaining life for prolonged periods of time when oral feedings are impossible or inadvisable, there is now exploration of the use of this type of parenteral feeding in the very small infant and in other infants who are ill and unable to tolerate oral feedings. Experience is limited at this point. This chapter can only suggest what is currently being done. The procedures, the fluids used and the route of administration probably will undergo rapid modification.

ROUTE OF ADMINISTRATION

The thoracic aorta, the inferior vena cava and peripheral scalp veins, entered with a no. 25 scalp vein needle, have all been used. We are not yet certain which method is most desirable. Certainly the delivery of hypertonic solutions into large-diameter vessels would seem to be safer than infusing these solutions into smaller vessels. We have treated some infants via the thoracic aorta and other infants via the superior vena cava, entering the latter by way of the jugular vein. We have not had sufficient experience to recommend a specific route of administration at this point.

FLUIDS AND EQUIPMENT

The ingredients listed in Table 15-1 are as satisfactory as any available at this time. We ask our pharmacy to use the strictest aseptic technics

Table 15-1. COMPOSITION OF PEDIATRIC
HYPERALIMENTATION SOLUTION

77 ml. of 50% dextrose plus 123 ml. of 5% Amigen with 5% dextrose; 1 ml. contains 1 calorie. 38.5 ml. of 50% dextrose plus 61.5 ml. of 5% Amigen with 5% dextrose.

The following are the electrolyte concentrations (mEq./100 ml.): sodium 2.15, potassium 1.17, calcium 0.31, magnesium 0.12, chloride 1.23 and phosphate 1.35.

The pH of the solution without buffering is 5.0. Thus we have added variable amounts of sodium bicarbonate to the solution, as follows: 5 ml. $NaHCO_3$ added to 200 ml. of solution raises the ph to 6.6; 7.5 ml., to 6.7; 12.5 ml., to 7.0; and 15.0 ml., to 7.0.

Note

For the newborn infant and the very low-birthweight infant a diluted solution (0.33 cal./ml. to 0.50 cal./ml.) should be used, if it is started early, before extreme weight loss occurs. It can then be concentrated further, according to tolerance.

in preparing the solution. Undoubtedly improvements will be made in the next few years in the composition of high-caloric intravenous solutions.

The volume of parenteral fluid may start as low as 60 ml./kg. per day and may be increased to as much as 120 ml./kg. per day. The desirable strength of the solution is not yet specifically known. We have used 65-120 cal./100 ml. (1 cal./ml.), and have not noticed any difference in the response or intolerance. In excess of 1 cal./ml., glucosuria is detected.

The fluids should be placed in a volumetric flask and delivered to the patient through sterile tubing, at the end of which a 0.22-micron Millipore filter removes bacterial and particulate matter. One must be sure to obtain the correct filter, because some are available with considerably larger pores. All of the tubing up to the umbilical catheter or to the scalp vein exit should be changed at least every 24 hours, and we may need to recommend more frequent changes.

DURATION OF THERAPY

Obviously this type of therapy should not be long continued. In infants who have intact gastrointestinal tracts, 10% glucose is given orally very early, and the amount is increased until the infant is able to tolerate 80-100 ml./kg. per day, orally; then the parenteral fluids are discontinued. If the gastrointestinal tract cannot accept fluids (as in a postoperative ileal resection for ileal atresia), parenteral fluids may need to be considered for a longer period of time. The maximum length of time we have left an umbilical artery catheter in place is 26 days, and no complications developed.

One untested and undocumented method of delivering high-caloric fluids to infants is to give a fat-rich meal to a prospective donor and then take 500 ml. of blood from this donor. The serum is separated and the cells are retransfused to the donor. The serum is broken into small packs and delivered to the infant daily or on alternate days.

PROCEDURES

After the infant's requirements have been calculated, the infusion can begin. We start with one-half the patient's actually calculated need. Over several days' time we increase the amounts, trying to obtain the projected target. Tables 15-2 and 15-3 suggest the main nutritional requirements.

During this time several values must be watched. Electrolytes, daily for 3-4 days, may be necessary; however, electrolyte imbalance has not been a significant problem. The urinary glucose should be monitored by Clinitest; if the values, obtained four times daily, are a mixture of +3 and +4 we decrease the amount of solution being infused. Quantities of urinary sugars can be tested also; if more than 1.5% of the glucose being infused arrives in the urine, one should decrease the solute load. And, of course, blood urea nitrogen and the infant's weight should be monitored.

Obviously, this is a high solute load; if the osmotic load becomes too large, then rapid weight loss can occur. Thus, daily weights should be checked.

The physician should be watchful for the following known side effects of hyperalimentation: hyperglycemia, glycosuria with osmotic diuresis and dehydration, reactive hypoglycemia, superior vena cava obstruction, and infection.

Table 15-2. NUTRITIONAL REQUIREMENTS OF INFANTS

Nutrient	Orally	Intravenously
Protein (gm./kg.)	3	4-6
Calories per Kilogram	60-120	130-35
Water (ml./kg.)	150	150
Chloride (mEq./kg.)	8	2-5
Sodium (mEq./kg.)	8	4-5
Potassium (mEq./kg.)	8	4-5
Calcium (mEq./kg.)	12	4
Phosphorus (mEq./kg.)	7	4-6
Magnesium (mEq./kg.)	5	1.5-2.0

Table 15-3. VITAMIN REQUIREMENTS OF INFANTS

Vitamin	Orally	Intravenously
A	1,500 IU	3000 IU
Thiamine	0.4 mg.	15 mg.
Riboflavin	0.6 mg.	3 mg.
Pyridioxine	0.25 mg.	4.5 mg.
C	30 mg.	150 mg.
D	400 IU	300 IU
E	--	1.5 IU
Niacin	6 mg.	30 mg.
Folic acid	0.35 mg.	0.5 mg.
K	1.5 mg.	1 mg.

SUGGESTED READINGS

1. Auld, P. A. M., Bhangananda, P., and Mehta, S.: The influence of an early caloric intake with intravenous glucose on catabolism of premature infants, Pediatrics 37:592, 1966.
2. Cornblath, M., Forbes, A. E., Pildes, R., and Greengard, J.: A controlled study of early fluid administration on survival of low birth weight infants (abst.), Proc. 76th Am. Meeting, Am. Pediat. Soc. 1966, p. 14.
3. Garrow, J. S., and Pike, M. C.: The long-term prognosis of severe infantile malnutrition, Lancet 1:1, 1967.

4. Gerda, I. M., Beuda, M. D., and Babson, S. G.: Peripheral intravenous alimentation of the small premature infant, J. Pediat. 79:494, 1971.

5. Wilmore, D. W., Groft, B. D., Bishop, H. C., and Dudrick, S. J.: Total parenteral nutrition in infants with catastrophic gastrointestinal anomalies, J. Pediat. Surg. 4:181, 1969.

APPENDIX 1

Miscellaneous Routines and Orders

ROUTINE NEWBORN ORDERS

A. Transitional nursery
1. Admit to transitional nursery, in infant warmer.
2. NPO for 6 hr., then 3 oz. water every 4 hr. times 1 or 2 feedings, then formula, 3-4 oz. every 3-4 hr.
3. Temperature, pulse, respiration every 4 hr.
4. Dextrostix at age 1 hr.; repeat hourly until stable.
5. $AgNo_3$ drops 2 into each eye; irrigate with saline.
6. Aquamephyton, 1 mg, IM, times 1.
7. If stable, transfer to normal nursery at 24 hr.

B. Term, nonrisk infants
1. Transfer to normal nursery; continue above orders except: temperature, pulse, respiration every 12 hr.
2. Alcohol to cord every 12 hr.
3. Circumcise, with parental permission.

C. Risk infants (Less than 2,500 Gm., infants of toxemic mothers, infants of diabetic mothers, infants born by c-section, small-for-date babies).
1. Place in Isolette. No O_2 unless cyanotic. If cyanotic may give O_2 without physician's order. Isolette temp. at $90°F$. until baby's temperature reaches $97°$, then reduce to $86°$. If baby's temperature is less than $92°$, set Isolette at $94°$. Humidity 60%.
2. NPO until ordered.
3. See specific section.

D. Isolette. The following infants should be placed in Isolettes:
1. Less than 2,500 Gm. (5½ lb).
2. Greater than 4,175 Gm. (9 lb); potential diabetic mother.
3. Infants of diabetics.

4. Infants of toxemics.
5. C-sections.
6. Babies with Apgar less than 6 at 1 or 5 minutes.
7. Infants admitted from outside the hospital.
8. Any sick infant.

E. Isolation
   1. Because the Isolette is an isolation unit it is not necessary to put babies in Isolettes in isolation.
   2. Unsterile or outborn infants may be put either in Isolettes or observation nursery.

LOW-BIRTHWEIGHT INFANTS: SUGGESTED PROCEDURES 0-72 HOURS

A. General
   1. Pediatric staff or house officer should attend all deliveries when any problem anticipated.
   2. All infants will be placed in an Isolette on their backs, with shoulders slightly elevated and head extended, until feeding begins.
   3. Temperature of infants should be maintained as near 98.6° (R) or 97.6° (Ax) as possible by Isolette adjustment, radiant heat, wrapping extremities, etc.
   4. Humidity should be kept at 60%.
   5. No antibiotics unless specifically indicated.

B. Infants 1,200-2,000 Gm.
   1. Institute oral glucose (10%) at *3 hours* of age, 5-30 ml./hr., depending on size.
   2. Dilute formula (5-10 cal./oz.) may be instituted after 1 or 2 water feedings.
   3. Further increase as tolerated so that by 5th day infant is receiving 150 ml./kg. of water and by 8th day 125 cal./kg.
   4. Vitamin C, 50 mg., 1st day PO or IM, thereafter 0.6 ml. Tri-Vi-Sol daily.
   5. Begin Fer-In-Sol 0.3 ml. to 0.6 ml. daily at 10 days to 2 weeks.
   6. Keep in Isolette until approximately 2,000 Gm.

7. Hct. weekly or oftener.
8. Dextrostix frequently (about every 3 hr.) until stable.

C. Infants less than 1,200 Gm. (0-72 hours)
1. Insert arterial and/or venous umbilical catheter as soon after birth as possible; obtain pH and serum K stat, and P_{O_2}, P_{CO_2}.
2. If pH is greater than 7.3 and no hyperkalemia, begin parenteral 5 or 10% glucose, 60 ml./kg./day.
3. If pH is less than 7.3, add to the glucose as follows:

pH	NaHCO$_3$
7.2-7.3	5 mEq./100 ml. glucose
7.1-7.2	10 mEq./100 ml. glucose
7.0-7.1	15 mEq./100 ml. glucose
Less than 7.0	25 mEq./100 ml. glucose

pH should be corrected in 6 hours. Additional amounts of NaHCO$_3$ (5 mEq.) may be given by intra-arterial push.
4. If serum K is greater than 8.0 mg%, or between 6.0-8.0 mg% with bradycardia, precede NaHCO$_3$ with 10% glucose plus insulin (1 unit/3 gm. glucose) until symptoms regress.
5. Oxygen: give enough to keep infant pink, or 60-80 mm. Hg PaO$_2$. Consider assisted ventilation or continuous positive airway pressure (see Chap. 5) after above therapy if:

   a. There are repeated and prolonged apneic spells.
   b. Gases: P_{CO_2} > 70 mm Hg
      PaO$_2$ < 40 mm Hg
      pH < 7.2
   c. Silverman Score < 6

	0	1	2
Cyanosis	0	mild	severe
Retraction	0	minimal	marked
Grunting	0	stethoscope	hear without scope
Breath sounds	0	fair exchange	no exchange
Resp. rate	0	60-80	< 40- >80

6. Place under bilirubin reduction lamp if serum bilirubin exceeds 10 mg% (indirect).

HYALINE MEMBRANE SYNDROME

A. Risk Infants: low birthweight, toxemic mothers, diabetic mothers, c-section.

B. Recognition: expiratory grunt, tachypnea, retractions, all with or without cyanosis should institute diagnostic studies.

C. Diagnosis and treatment
   1. Baby is presumably in Isolette, on back, shoulders elevated, head extended, receiving O_2 if cyanotic.
   2. Insert radiopaque no. 5 catheter into umbilical artery (if unsuccessful use umbilical vein).
   3. Withdraw blood for arterial pH, P_{O_2}, K^+ (give O_2 to keep baby pink or keep PaO_2 40-70 mm.Hg).
   4. Inject 5 mEq. $NaHCO_3$ into artery over a 5-minute period.
   5. Run arterial drip of 5-10% glucose (60 ml./kg./day).
   6. *Obtain chest x-ray to:*
      a. Exclude surgically treatable lesions (emphysema, pneumothorax, etc.).
      b. Exclude pneumonia.
      c. Assure that arterial catheter is in aorta or, if in vein, in vena cava.
      d. If a. and b. are excluded, the infant is treated for hyaline membrane syndrome.
   7. Therapy with 5-10% glucose continues at 60-150 ml./kg./day plus $NaHCO_3$ added as described under prematures 0-72 hours. The pH should be corrected in 6 hours; P_{O_2} should be 60-80 mm.Hg. If excess $NaHCO_3$ (more than 15 mEq.) is needed in the first 6 hours THAM may be given, but not in umbilical vein.
   8. No antibiotics unless infant becomes worse or has not improved in 24-48 hours.
   9. Artificial ventilatory assistance as indicated (see section on premature).
   10. Repeat x-ray if condition deteriorates.

11. Discontinuance of parenteral fluids and institution of oral feeds depends on infant's progress.

SEPTICEMIA

A. No "prophylactic" antibiotics are used. When given, they are given in therapeutic doses.

B. There are actually three types of sepsis of the newborn:
  1. Prenatal: rubella, CMI, etc.
  2. Intranatal: acquired secondarily to amniotic infection, usually following premature membrane rupture. Sick at birth.
  3. Postnatal (2-3 days of age). Acquired from personnel or other babies; usually coliform organisms.

C. Recognition
  1. Before and at birth: signs of maternal infections, fetal tachycardia, infant or amniotic fluid smells bad, early respiratory distress. THESE BABIES SHOULD BE CULTURED AND TREATED.
  2. Later onset.
     a. Constant signs: "looks ill, refuses food, vomits"
     b. Common signs: jaundice, respiratory distress, fever, hypothermia, lethargy, apnea, cyanosis, diarrhea, etc. These babies should be cultured; institution of therapy is a matter of clinical judgment.

D. Diagnosis. Prior to institution of therapy, the following cultures should be obtained:
  1. Throat.
  2. Rectum.
  3. Blood.
  4. Urine (suprapubic aspiration).
  5. Spinal fluid.
  6. External ear.
  7. Examine gastric contents for PMN.

E. Therapy
  1. Ampicillin 100 mg./kg./day IV or IM times 5 days.

2. Kanamycin 7-15 mg./kg./day IM, 2 divided doses, 5 days.
3. Change to more specific antibiotics if indicated by sensitivities.

INFANTS OF TOXEMIC MOTHERS

A. If mother has received any antihypertensives or if infant is depressed at birth, he should be placed in Isolette for 24 hr.

B. Dextrostix should be monitored every 6 hrs. especially from 48 to 72 hr. Rx hypoglycemia as below.

C. If $MgSO_4$ has been given to mothers, cord Mg should be obtained.

INFANTS OF DIABETIC MOTHERS
(Gestational, Insulin-Dependent, and Babies who weigh over 9 lb.)

A. All should be observed in an Isolette for at least 24 hr., longer if ill.

B. Primary observations are for hypoglycemia and hypocalcemia.

C. Procedures
   1. Dextrostix should be done at 0, 30 min., 60, 90, 120, then hourly until age 12 hr.
   2. If the blood glucose drops below 40 mg%, oral 10% glucose should be given stat, 2-3 oz. If there is no prompt response, parenteral glucose should be given as outlined below.
   3. If infant's glucose remains normal, he should still begin oral 10% glucose at about 3 hr. of age as tolerated.
   4. If neuromuscular irritability or seizures develop the following should be done:
      a. Catheterize umbilical artery.
      b. Withdraw serum calcium sample.
      c. Give intra-arterially 1 Gm./kg. of glucose (in 15-20% concentration) and 2 ml. of 10% calcium gluconate. Follow with 60 ml./kg./day, 10% glucose drip.
      d. Above may be repeated 1 or 2 times. When hypoglycemia persists, hydrocortisone may be given (10-15 mg./kg./day X 10 days).
      e. Other pharmacologic agents such as epinephrine should still be considered experimental.

HEMOLYTIC DISEASE OF NEWBORN

I. Laboratory protocol
   A. Problem: mother Rh- and father Rh+
      1. Do fetal blood group and Rh. If baby Rh neg., do direct
         Coombs; if negative, *STOP*
      2. If baby Rh+ do Coombs *stat.*
         a. If *Coombs-negative,* call pediatrician *promptly and stop.*
         b. If *Coombs-positive,* do cord bilirubin, *stat,* call pediatri-
            cian promptly.
   B. Problem: positive antibody screen.
      Proceed as above but do bilirubin only if ordered by pediatrician.

II. Indications for exchange transfusion in a Coombs-positive infant
    A. Hydrops fetalis: stat exchange (modified).
    B. Hct less than 45% with edema: stat exchange.
    C. Serum bilirubinemia according to Diamond's graph.
    D. Previous history of kernicterus or hydrops fetalis.

III. Exchange transfusion technic
     1. Standard technic, in Isolette or under Infawarmer, with
        type–specific RhO–blood compatible with mother.
     2. Preparation should include:
        a. Emptying the stomach and leaving tube in place.
        b. Attaching a cardiac monitor or stethoscope to the chest.
        c. Four ml./lb. of salt-poor human albumin may be given
           30-45 min. prior to exchange when exchange is being
           done for hyperbilirubinemia. We do not do this regularly.
     3. The remainder of the technic is standard.
        a. The increments used (10-20 ml. of blood) depend on the
           infant's size and condition.
        b. If two operators are present, the procedure may be done
           by using the vein and artery.
        c. At least a one volume exchange should be done.
        d. One ml. of 10% calcium gluconate should be given slowly
           through the umbilical catheter every 100 ml.
        e. Venous pressure should not exceed 10 mm. Hg and should
           be measured at the beginning and at each 100-ml.
           interval.

    f. Although one should begin with a 20-ml. deficit, this deficit should be corrected at the conclusion, if the venous pressure is less than 10 mm. Hg.

IV. ABO Incompatibility. When therapy is required, is essentially the same as above.

Pharmacopeia

A list of drugs frequently used in the newborn infant, with route of administration, dosage and special hazards, follows. For a more detailed pharmacopeia the reader is referred to Schaeffer, A. S. and Avery, M. E.: *Diseases of the Newborn* (3d ed.; Philadelphia: W. B. Saunders Company, 1971), pp. 871-877.

DRUG	ROUTE & DOSAGE	SPECIAL HAZARDS
Albumin	IV, 0.5-1.0 Gm./kg.	Calculate need based on plasma volume and TSP.
Ampicillin	IV, IM, 100-400 mg./kg./day, divided doses every 4 hr. IV, every 8 hr. IM	
Blood	IV, packed cells 5-10 ml./kg. IV, whole cells 10 ml./kg.	Calculate need based on hct., blood volume and desired hct.
Calcium gluconate 9% calcium	IV, 0.5-1.0 Gm./kg./ day 2-4 ml. per injection	Bradycardia, irritating to tissues
Calcium lactate	PO 0.5 mg./kg./day	
Cortisone	PO 5-15 mg./kg./day	
Desoxycorticosterone Acetate (DOCA)	IM, 1-5mg./day as required	
Digoxin	IV, IM, 0.03-0.05 mg./kg. total digitalizing dose, ½ stat, remainder in 2 doses at 6-8 hr. intervals; maintenance ¼-½ total dose	

DRUG	ROUTE & DOSAGE	SPECIAL HAZARDS
Epinephrine	1:1,000 subcutaneous, 0.05 mg. (dilute)	Local vasoconstriction
Gentamicin	IV, IM, 3-7 mg./kg./day	Special precaution in anuria
Glucagon	IM, IV, 30-100 μg./kg. every 6-12 hr.	
Heparin	IV, 100 U/kg./4-6 hr.	Intractable bleeding
Insulin	IV, IM, 0.1-1.0 U/kg.	For transient hyperglycemia
Kanamycin	IM, 7-15 mg./kg./day in 2-3 doses	Nephrotoxic, ototoxic
Mercuhydrin	IV, 0.25-0.50 ml. every other day	
Methcillin (staphcillin)	IV, IM, 100-200 mg./kg./day	
NaHCO$_3$	IV, empirically 2-4 mEq./kg., otherwise according to pH	
Penicillin	IV, IM, 50,000 U/kg.	
Phenobarbital	PO, IM, 8-10 mg./kg.	
Plasma	IV, 20 ml./kg.	
Thyroid Extract	PO, 0.015 Gm./day	
Valium	IV, 0.1 mg. every 2-20 min. up to 1 mg.	
Vitamin B$_6$ (pyridoxine)	PO, IV, 5 mg./day	
Vitamin C (ascorbic acid)	PO, 25-50 mg./day	
Vitamin K	IM, PO, 1-2 mg., 1 dose	

APPENDIX 3

Screening Procedures

The following procedures should be done on *all* infants:

A. Congenital anomaly appraisal (at birth)
   1. Inquire about polyhydramnios.
   2. Inspect abdomen for concavity.
   3. Pass nasal catheter bilaterally and nasogastric tube unilaterally.
   4. Aspiration of stomach contents; record amount and color.
   5. Insert rectal catheter and/or finger.
   6. Count umbilical arteries.

B. Urine examination for reducing substance (after 48-72 hr. milk) to exclude galactosemia, etc.

C. Guthrie test for phenylketonuria (after 48-72 hr. of milk feedings)

D. Hematocrit (PVC) within first hour of life

APPENDIX 4

Special Tests

A. Test for blood glucose<40 mg% with Dextrostix
   1. If Dextrostix<40 mg%, proceed.
   2. Do hematocrit. Put serum on Dextrostix.
   3. Wait 3 min.; wash with 20% (1/5 N) NaOH.
      a. No color change=20 mg%.
      b. Orange=20-30 mg%.
      c. Deep orange=30-40 mg%.

B. Apt test for swallowed blood syndrome
   1. Rinse blood with enough water to give pink color.
   2. To 5 ml. of the pink blood solution add 1 ml. 0.25 N (1%) NaOH.
   3. Do known control also and compare.

University of Nebraska College of Medicine Department of Nursing Service

PROCEDURES FOR ENTERING NURSERY

I. Nursing service personnel, nursing students and faculty
   1. Go to nurses' lounge and change into a short-sleeved scrub dress. Hair must be off collar and out of face—neat.
   2. Remove all jewelry, except plain wedding bands.
   3. Enter nursery and wash hands and arms to elbow with provided soap.
   4. Scrub hands and wash arms to elbow, using brush and antibacterial soap, for 3 minutes.
   5. *Wash hands again between handling each baby.*

II. Other authorized personnel
   Staff and resident physician
   Student physician (M/4 and M/3)
   Delivery room personnel
   Laboratory technicians
   X-ray technicians
   1. Remove all jewelry.
   2. Don long-sleeved gown if baby is to be held.
   3. Scrub hands, using brush and antibacterial soap for 3 minutes, in nursing station.
   4. Enter nursery.
   5. Wash hands again between handling each baby.

ADMISSION OF NEWBORN INFANT

Infants are brought to the nursery from the delivery room. Delivery and nursery personnel check the weight together. The identification of infant should be checked by nursery nurse. The following applies only to routine newborn care. Specific orders will be given for sick or premature infants.

1. Place the infant in heated crib.
2. Nursery personnel wash hands.
3. Observe infant's general appearance, especially for cyanosis or hemorrhage. Note infant's color, activity, respirations, type of cry and heart rate.
4. Take quiet respiratory rate for *one full minute.* If respirations are above 60 or below 25/min., notify pediatric resident.
5. Check cord stump for bleeding on admission.
6. Check respiration and cord stumps every 30 minutes X 3.
7. Temperature, respiratory rate and cord stump are checked again at 4 and 8 hours.
8. All infants are to have a bath on admission, using an antibacterial soap.
9. Place in warmer, or under heat lamp, on side or abdomen.
10. Mark infant's unit with a crib card.
11. Chart observations accurately on chart and work sheet.
12. Infant may go to mother when mother's and infant's condition are stable. The unwed mother may see, hold and feed infant if she wishes.
13. Put silver nitrate in eyes.
14. Give Aquamephyton 1 mg. IM.
15. Do hematocrit if medical students are not available.

NORMAL NEWBORN NURSERY

1. Baths are done daily in the A.M. Use soap sparingly; if skin is dry do not use soap at all except on the baby's bottom.
2. Use the bath basins in the cribs. All necessary items should be stocked.
3. When weighing the babies check with the previous day's weight and if there is a 100 Gm. difference, reweigh the baby and have a second person double check.
4. Cribs should be stocked with soap, lotion, washcloth, cotton balls and a comb. Linens should include 4-6 cloth diapers,

1-1½ dozen disposable diapers, 2-4 crib sheets, 4-6 shirts and 4-6 blankets. Try and keep girls in pink and boys in blue. These are to be checked at the end of each shift.
5. The baby and the crib should be kept clean and dry!
6. The crib cards are to be filled out completely. Check these at the beginning of your shift as you take the babies out. Extra information to be put in the right-hand corner includes the status of the mother as to keeping and whether or not she is feeding or nursing.
7. A clean wrapper is to be used each time the baby is handled. Babies are not to be held, except in cases of emergency, without a wrapper.
8. Any babies fed in the nursery are to be held, not propped.

CIRCUMCISIONS

1. The responsibility of obtaining the permit is the post partum ward clerk's or other personnel's.
2. Circumcisions are done by the obstetric intern or resident on the second day of life.
3. Premature infants are circumcised at 5 days if condition permits.
4. Be sure there is an order and a permit.
5. The charge nurse is to notify the intern or resident in the A.M.
6. After the circumcision the baby is to be diapered and placed on his side and checked every 15 minutes for 1 hour for bleeding. The first voiding should be charted as such.
7. Do not remove the dressing.

TRANSITIONAL NURSERY

All new babies are to go to this nursery and be placed in a warmer or an Isolette for 24 hours—the exception being prematures, who go to the intensive care nursery.

Guidelines for this nursery:
1. Baby may be taken to mother for her to see in 4 hours, if baby is stable.

2. Give baby first feeding of sterile water in 6 hours. Feed in nursery.
3. At the next regular feeding time, give 5% glucose water.
   Baby may go to mother at next feeding for formula or breast.
4. New baby is to stay in warmer or Isolette for 24 hours.
   Exceptions:
   a. If you need a warmer for a new baby and all are in use, move oldest infant, providing baby is stable.
   b. Doctor writes orders to move earlier or stay longer.
5. Baby may go to mother for feedings (starting with third) while in warmer for 24 hours.

EYE TREATMENT AFTER DELIVERY

I. Purpose
   A. Prophylactic treatment of the eyes for gonorrhea.

II. Equipment
   A. Ampoule silver nitrate 1%.
   B. Needle.
   C. Ampoule sterile water.
   D. Medicine dropper.
   E. Cotton balls.

III. Procedure
   A. Cleanse eyes with cotton balls with eyes closed.
   B. Pierce end of ampoule of silver nitrate with needle.
   C. Break sterile water ampoule and draw enough sterile water to irrigate eyes.
   D. Separate eyelids and instill 2 drops silver nitrate; leave for ½ minute or longer.
   E. Irrigate eye with sterile water.
   F. Repeat D and E for other eye.
      Eye-dropper wrapper can be used as a sterile field.

DAILY NURSERY JOBS

1. Each shift is to stock cribs, Isolettes and cupboards.
2. The emergency cart is to be checked and restocked by each shift.

3. Isolettes are to be changed weekly.
4. Oxygen tubing is to be changed every 24 hours. This includes humidifiers.
5. IV tubing is to be changed every 24 hours.
6. Water is to be changed in the Isolettes every 24 hours.
7. Suction bulb and cup are to be changed every 2-3 days.
8. Suction tubing is to be changed every 24 hours.

DAILY CARE, INTENSIVE CARE UNIT

1. Take vital signs every 4 hours; if abnormal take oftener.
2. Bathe only if condition permits. Use soap sparingly; pat, do not rub.
3. Weigh Monday and Thursday unless otherwise ordered.
4. Clean cord with soap and water as well as with 70% alcohol twice a day even if catheter is indwelling.
5. Keep infant on abdomen and sides when condition permits. If on back have small roll under shoulders.
6. Measure head and length weekly.
7. Check oxygen every 2-4 hours, depending on condition.
8. Monitor leads are to be changed and rotated every 8 hours or every 24 hours depending on size of infant and condition of skin.
9. Small infants receive Tri-Vi-Sol, 0.6 ml. if on oral feeding, 25 mg. vitamin C IM if N.P.O.
10. Fer-In-Sol 0.3 ml.; 0.6 ml. is started on the 10th to 14th day, depending on size.

INITIAL WATER

I. Purpose
   A. To check sucking reflex.
   B. To check patent esophagus.
   C. To loosen mucus, so it can be regurgitated more easily.

II. Equipment
   A. Infant that has orders written for initial water, usually 6 hours of age.

B. Sterile H_2O

C. Disposable diaper for bubbling.

D. Wrapper.

III. Procedure

A. Check infant to make sure he is clean and dry.

B. Wrap infant according to wrapper technic.

C. Hold infant upright and give water.

D. While giving water check:

    1. Sucking reflex.

    2. Amount of mucus.

    3. Esophageal patency.

    4. Regurgitation.

    5. Cyanosis, etc.

E. Unwrap infant and place in crib on abdomen or side.

IV. Recording

A. Information to be charted:

    1. Time and amount of water taken.

    2. Type of sucking reflex.

    3. Amount of mucus.

    4. Regurgitation.

    5. Anything unusual noted.

FEEDING

I. Purpose

A. To make the entire procedure a satisfying experience for the mother and the baby.

II. Equipment

A. Bottle with formula or water for each baby.

B. Disposable diaper for bubbling.

III. Procedure

A. Babies fed by mothers

    1. Prepare formula or water.

    2. Check with charge nurse if there is any question as to whether or not the baby is to go to the mother.

3. WASH HANDS WELL BETWEEN BABIES!
4. Make sure baby is clean and dry.
5. Wrap babies, using wrapper technics, and carry one at a time.
6. Be sure hand or breast care has been done before giving the baby to the mother.
7. Call the mother's name and check the Identabands.
8. For mother breast feeding
   a. Place the baby on his side so the tongue is parallel with the mother's nipple.
   b. See that the baby is always awake and nursing before leaving the bedside.
9. For mother bottle feeding
   a. Mother must be sitting in an upright position in bed or in a chair. She should be wearing a hospital gown.
   b. Place the baby in the mother's arms so that both are comfortable.
   c. Remove the cap from the bottle and make sure the milk is flowing. Instruct the mother to tilt bottle up so formula completely fills the nipple and lower portion of bottle, so that the baby will obtain less air.
10. General instructions to give the mother
    a. Keep the baby covered.
    b. Prevent contamination of the nipple.
    c. How to bubble the baby.
    d. How to keep the breast tissue from covering the baby's face.
    e. How to keep the baby awake.
    f. How to remove the nipple from the baby's mouth.
    g. How to get the baby to nurse.
    h. How long the baby should nurse (routine outline in procedure manual).
    i. How much formula to feed the infant.
11. Upon returning to the nursery, check to see if baby is clean and dry; place on abdomen or side. Check baby periodically to make sure infant is all right.

12. Recording
    a. Time, amount and how feeding was taken.
    b. Any problems connected with feeding.
    c. Be sure necessary information is in workbook.

B. Infants fed in the nursery
  1. Prepare ordered formula or water.
  2. Check with nurse in charge if any question as to whether baby should be fed.
  3. WASH HANDS BETWEEN EACH BABY!
  4. Wrap babies, using wrapper technic.
  5. All babies are to be held. ABSOLUTELY NO PROPPING!
  6. 20 minutes is sufficient time for feeding. If baby continually eats poorly in this amount of time ask the doctor for a gavage order.
  7. Bubble as often as seems necessary.
  8. Be sure baby is clean and dry before placing on side or abdomen in crib.
  9. Check several times between feedings to be sure baby is doing well.
  10. Record time and amount taken and any problems connected with feeding.

PRECAUTIONS IN FEEDING

1. Don't overtax the infant's capacity for intake; this may lead to distention and regurgitation.
2. Sufficient allotment of time should be provided for feeding and burping. Avoid hurried procedures.
3. Vomiting, regurgitation, distention, fatigue or reflex attacks of apnea or cyanosis should be immediately reported to the physician.
4. The nurse should use discretion in situations where individual feedings may need to be interrupted or omitted entirely. This should be reported to the physician. Decisions concerning subsequent feedings are then made by him after he examines the infant and reviews the feeding history.

    5. Infants fed by nipple should be allowed to rest occasionally during the feeding. Actual feeding time should not exceed 20 minutes.

    6. When it is possible larger convalescing infants should be held and cuddled during the feeding.

MORNING CARE AND INSPECTION OF THE NEWBORN

I. Purpose
  A. To inspect infant for lesions and signs of infection and to make him clean and comfortable.
  B. To ascertain the infant's weight.
  C. To ascertain the infant's temperature.
  D. To obtain a picture of growth and development.

II. Equipment
  A. Nursery bath basin bundle.
  B. Thermometer.
  C. Antibacterial soap.
  D. Scale paper.
  E. Amphojel and cold cream.
  F. Rath scales.
  G. Linen.
    1. In bedside table.
    2. Each shift check supply and stock.
  H. Laundry hamper.
  I. Covered diaper can.
  J. Covered waste container.

III. Procedure
  A. Prepare field.
    1. Wash hands thoroughly.
    2. Obtain bath basin, thermometer and disposable diaper.
      a. Place contents (3 applicators, 2 cotton balls, 2 disposable washcloths) on disposable diaper.
      b. Fill basin 1/3 full of warm tap water. Place all equipment on disposable diaper on bedside table.

B. Bathe.
1. Cleanse eyes.
   a. Inspect eyes for discharge.
   b. Tear cotton ball in two parts and moisten in warm water.
   c. Use one part for each eye.
   d. Wipe gently from the inner canthus outward. Discard cotton ball.
   e. Tear remaining cotton ball in two parts and dry each eye.
2. Wash face with moistened cloth; dry.
3. Wash head, rinse and dry.
4. Unpin diaper, close pins and place on bedside table.
5. Take temperature. Put used thermometer on diaper on bedside table.
6. Remove shirt and diaper; place at lower end of crib.
7. Inspect upper part of body closely.
8. Wash upper body on 2d newborn day, and daily thereafter. Presently we are using clear water.
9. Wash premature infants as condition permits.
10. Always rinse thoroughly if soap is used.
11. Cleanse cord twice a day with soap, water and alcohol. Remove clamp when cord is dry.
12. Cleanse and rinse lower abdomen, legs, labia, groin and buttocks after each diaper change.
13. Discard soiled diaper in diaper can.

C. Clean crib.
1. Loosen diaper and crib sheet.
2. Pick baby up in crib sheet and cradle in arms.
3. Moisten corner of diaper at head of crib in bath basin and clean crib.

D. Weigh baby.
1. Take baby to scale in crib sheet.
2. Cover scale with scale paper.
3. Grasp baby's ankles with one hand, placing index finger between ankles. Support head, shoulders and back with other

hand and wrist, placing little finger in baby's axillary region.

   4. Place baby on scale.

E. Remove baby from the scale.

   1. Turn baby on abdomen.

   2. Place crib sheet over baby.

   3. Placé hands at sides of body, lift off scale and cradle in left arm.

   4. Discard paper. If necessary, clean scale tray.

   5. Return baby to crib after placing clean bed sheet in the bed.

F. Dress the baby.

   1. Place diaper under buttocks.

   2. Adjust diaper and pin, *point toward the back.* (Have fingers between baby and diaper when pinning.)

   3. Put on shirt, one sleeve at a time.

      a. Nurse puts her thumb and two fingers through sleeve, grasps baby's hand and pulls through sleeve.

      b. Secure ties.

      c. Fold shirt up even with edge of diaper.

      d. Cover hands.

G. Cover top 8 inches of mattress with clean diaper, to protect baby's face.

H. Cover with blanket, turning upper edge out and down if length permits. (Obtain clean blanket from cupboard if necessary and discard the soiled one.)

I. Clean table.

   1. Discard soiled linen in proper containers; e.g., place shirt in bag on side of hamper.

J. Empty bath basin.

K. Chart.

   1. Record on the chart board: weight, temperature, condition of eyes, skin, cord, buttocks, stool, voiding and any other symptom noted in columns.

L. After A.M. inspections are finished, wash and dry bath basins, take trays to delivery work room and put on central-supply cart.

DIAPERING

I. Purpose
  A. To keep infant clean, dry and comfortable.
  B. To prevent excoriated buttocks.

II. Equipment
  A. Disposable diapers.
  B. Washcloths.
  C. Any ordered medication.

III. Procedure
  A. WASH HANDS!
  B. Moisten washcloth and cleanse diaper area after all voidings and stools.
  C. Turn upper fold of blanket in and bring to foot of crib.
  D. Place infant on back, remove diaper and place CLOSED pins on top of work table.
  E. Wash area and dry well. Do this gently.
    1. Pay special attention to groin and, on males, around scrotum.
    2. On females cleanse from the vaginal area downward.
  F. Place soiled linens on work table and cleanse this area when finished.
  G. If buttocks are red or excoriated:
    1. After cleansing do one of the following:
      a. Apply A & D, zinc oxide. No order is needed.
      b. Special medication if ordered.
      c. Expose area to air and heat by placing exposed buttocks to heat lamp placed 12-18 inches from the area.
      d. Notify nurse in charge.
  H. On male infants who have been circumcised, leave surgical or other dressings alone and cleanse by squeezing water from washcloth over area.
  I. Apply clean diaper. Fold plastic to the inside, both front and back, and pin below the umbilical cord with the pins toward the back.

GAVAGE PROCEDURE

I. Purpose
   To provide necessary fluid and caloric intake.

II. Equipment
   A. Formula.
   B. No. 5 or no. 8 feeding tube.
   C. Syringe.
   D. Stethoscope.
   E. Tape.

III. Procedure
   A. Oral Insertion
   1. Place a small roll under baby's neck, to help stabilize head.
   2. Measure from the mouth to just left of the umbilicus; mark with a piece of tape.
   3. Pass tube slowly through the mouth until the mark is reached, stopping and withdrawing tube if child gags, coughs or turns cyanotic.
   4. Secure with small piece of tape to chin.
   5. Attach syringe and insert several cc.s of air while listening with stethoscope over abdomen. (Swish will be heard.)
   6. Aspirate gently until no more stomach contents return. If contents mostly mucus, discard; if formula, return and subtract from total amount of formula given.
   7. Remove syringe from feeding tube and remove plunger.
   8. Attach syringe to feeding tube.
   9. Pour necessary amount of formula into syringe.
   10. Push gently to start flow.
   11. Allow formula to go in by gravity only. It may be necessary to give a slight push periodically.
   12. Continue to add formula until ordered amount is reached or baby begins pushing back and acting uncomfortable so that flow by gravity ceases.
   13. Remove syringe from tube; close end of tube.
   14. Remove tube quickly.
   15. Sit infant up and attempt to bubble.

16. Place on abdomen whenever possible.
17. Infant may need to be bubbled before end of feeding also.

B. Nasal insertion
  1. Measure from nose to ear to bottom of sternum; mark with a small piece of tape.
  2. Insert gently, moving head from side to side until tube passes easily. Aim tube parallel to the hard palate (greatest aperture).
  3. Secure with tape.
  4. Proceed same as oral.
  5. When feeding is completed, be sure end of feeding tube is closed.
  6. Flush tube with plain sterile H_2O.

C. Chart
  1. Amount and kind of feeding.
  2. Any difficulty with insertion of catheter.

CARE OF BABIES IN ISOLETTES

1. Take vital signs every 4 hours, more often if abnormal.
2. Bathe daily, using small amount of soap every other day or prn.
3. Pat when bathing; do not rub.
4. Weigh Monday and Thursday unless ordered otherwise. This is just for the babies in Isolettes.
5. Change linen as required. Do not put clean linen on top of dirty linen.
6. Clean cord with soap, followed with alcohol twice a day or as required. Use 70% alcohol only.
7. Keep baby on abdomen or side only, on abdomen at least 1 hour after feeding.
8. Measure premature infant's head and length once a week, in or out of Isolette.

OXYGEN

1. Oxygen is to be ordered by percentage, not by liters.
2. Check oxygen every 2 to 4 hours and record.
3. Check oxygen every ½ hour times 3 if concentration has been changed.
4. Oxygen should be used:
   a. In episodes of cyanosis—baby may need gentle suctioning. Give oxygen by mask, enough to overcome cyanosis. Up to 100% may be used.
   b. With gradual onset of cyanosis increase oxygen by 5% increments to relieve.
   c. Always inform physician whenever a. or b. occurs.
5. Crystals in oxygen analyzer should be blue, not lavender. They should be changed by whoever finds them lavender.

CARE OF ISOLETTES

1. Temperature should be regulated according to the needs of the baby.
2. Temperatures of the Isolette should be recorded and adjusted if baby's temperature is abnormal.
3. Ambient or incubator temperature should be kept below 94°F. and radiant heat used to supplement if baby's temperature is still low.
4. Humidity, unless ordered otherwise, should be kept halfway between maximum and minimum.
5. Change Isolette at least once a week.
6. Change water reservoir daily on the 11-7 shift. This includes the Isolettes that are warming.
7. Do not use alcohol on glass part of isolette.

MONITORS

A. Apnea monitors
   1. Skin should be clean and dry (including vernix caseosa).
   2. Apply disk over end of lead, leaving gray portion on.

3. Put Redux (or whatever gel is available) into center portion of lead.
4. Remove gray portion of disk.
5. Place on baby. Whenever possible put under the arms.
6. If necessary use small amount of tape to keep in place.
7. Turn monitor on. Alarm will go off for a few seconds.
8. Check to see if leads are on properly by turning dial to "Impedence." If it goes into the red area something is wrong; therefore it will be necessary to start over.
9. Adjust sensitivity.
10. If leads become loose, start all over again. DO NOT KEEP PUTTING TAPE OVER THE LEADS.

B. Cardiac monitors
   1. Application is the same as for the apnea monitor, with the following exceptions:
      a. Place leads on both arms and the left leg. The leads are marked.
      b. Set the high and low readings according to the doctor's orders.

C. Care of the monitors
   1. After use, soak the leads in normal saline. This helps to loosen all the gel. (This should be done every couple of days while in use.)
   2. If necessary, soak in a tape-removing solution.
   3. When monitors are discontinued, please wind up cords and place back in cupboards. This is to be done by whoever removes them from the baby.
   4. If monitors do not work properly, please notify the head nurse or supervisor.

This equipment is expensive and to work properly, it must have good care.

DEXTROSTIX PROCEDURE

A. Purpose
To measure the blood sugar by heel stick.

B. Equipment:
   1. Dextrostix
   2. Alco wipe
   3. Lancet
   4. Water
   5. Clock

C. Procedure
   1. Warm heel if time. Clean bottom of heel with Alco wipe.
   2. Milk foot from front to back. Avoid squeezing.
   3. Make small puncture. Lancet should go in at an angle.
   4. Milk foot from front to back to obtain a generous drop of blood on Dextrostix on filter side.
   5. Begin timing as soon as first drop is on Dextrostix. More blood may be added after timing starts.
   6. At EXACTLY 60 seconds, rinse with water.
   7. Match color with chart on bottle.
   8. Record and report abnormal readings to doctor in charge.

ROUTINE DOCTOR'S ORDERS

A. Term, nonrisk infants
   1. Admit to transitional nursery on abdomen and sides only.
   2. NPO for 6 hours, then sterile water X 1 or 2, then 5% glucose water X 1 or 2. Then formula or breast every 3-4 hours.
   3. Silver nitrates drops, 2 in each eye. Irrigate well with sterile water then and as required.
   4. 70% alcohol to cord twice a day.
   5. Aquamephyton 1 mg. I.M. X 1.
   6. Circumcision with permission on normal males.

B. Risk infants (Less than 2,500 Gm.; infants of toxemic, diabetic or sectioned mothers)
   1. Place in Isolette. No oxygen unless cyanotic. Isolette temperature at 90° until infant's temperature stabilizes; use extra lamps over Isolette. When temperature reaches 97°, reduce extra heat. Humidity 60%.
   2. NPO until ordered.

3. Notify physician on call immediately.

4. Eye drops and Aquamephyton same as above.

5. 25-50 mg. of vitamin C to all true premature infants. Continue on 25 mg. daily until infant feeds, then change to Tri-Vi-Sol .03 ml. every day. Orally, change to 0.6 ml. daily when infant begins to recover. Start Fer-In-Sol on 10th to 14th day, 0.6 ml.

Index

A

Abdomen
  cellulitis, and septicemia, 142
  inspection, 50
  variations from normal, 36
ABO incompatibility, 13
Achondroplasia, 71
Acidosis: and resuscitation
  failures, 47
Adenomatoid malformation:
  pulmonary, 90-91
Adrenal hyperplasia: virilizing,
  salt-losing type, 71
Adrenogenital syndrome, 70-71
Age (*see* Gestational age)
Agenesis: pulmonary, 89-90
Air transportation: of sick infant,
  226
Airway(s)
  anomalies, congenital, 47
  equipment for resuscitation,
  48
  upper, obstruction, 80-81
Alcohol: and hyperbilirubinemia, 101
Alimentation, total intravascular, 241-245
  administration route, 241
  equipment for, 241-242
  fluids for, 241-242
  procedures, 243-244
  therapy duration, 242-243
Amniocentesis: technic, 17-18
Amnionitis, 10
Amniotic fluid
  infection, causing pneumonia, 140

spectrophotometry of, 14
Anemia, 110-123
  blood loss, 117-120, 121
    clinical features, 118-119
    diagnosis, 119
    hematologic features, 118-119
    treatment, 120
  classification, 111
  after first day of life, 120-123
  hemolytic, nonspherocytic,
    122-123
  infection and, 121
Angiography: in congenital heart
  disease, 200-201
Ankle dorsiflexion: in gestational
  age estimation, 29
Anomalies, 49-79
  adenomatoid, pulmonary, 90-91
  airway, congenital, 47
  appraisal, 49-50
    outline of, 50
  central nervous system, 65
  chest, 59-62
  chromosomes causing, 73-77
  congenital, 47, 49-79
  extremities, 65-66
    upper, in newborn of diabetic
    mother, 72
  eye, 66-68
  head, 57-59
  incidence, 51
  intestine, 62-64
  requiring immediate attention,
    57-68
  requiring immediate surgery,
    57-68
  skin, 66, 72-73
  stomach, 62-64

PB-331-4
5-26
B-T

3 1222 00000 5507

NO LONGER THE PROPERTY
OF THE
UNIVERSITY OF R. I. LIBRARY